I'M TOUGHER THAN I LOOK

The Sue Miller Story

I'm Tougher Than I Look

The Sue Miller Story

As told to Amber Dahlin

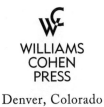

WILLIAMS COHEN PRESS

Denver, Colorado

Book layout and design by Margaret McCullough
Corvus Design Studio & Publishing Services
corvusdesignstudio.com

WILLIAMS
COHEN
PRESS

2400 Cherry Creek Drive South #209
Denver, CO 80209
U.S.A.

ISBN 1-59975-469-X

First Edition: April 2006
Printed and Bound in Canada

DEDICATION

I dedicate this book to Dr. Peter Mayerson,
who helped me come out
from underneath the couch!

ACKNOWLEDGMENTS

I THANK THE FOLLOWING PEOPLE:

- My children, their spouses, and my grandchildren for never leaving my side.
- Amber Dahlin for making sense of my tears and ramblings.
- Elise Spain for keeping the purpose of this book straight in my mind.
- My sister Judy and brother-in-law Arthur for always believing in me no matter what I did.
- My friends for their ongoing support through the years.

AMBER'S THANKS:

- Sally Shriner for pressure-cooker manuscript preparation.
- Susan Poulin, Cathleen Galitz and Steve Friedman for their Bestsellers attitude.
- Julie Zander, Connie Nelson, and Darlene Dahlin for thorough response.
- Corvus Publishing Group for manuscript design and project support.

TABLE OF CONTENTS

Foreword

A Way of Caring

By Linda Ellerbee

Sue Miller came into my life in 1993. In 1992, I had been diagnosed with breast cancer. I lost both my breasts and all my hair.

My hair grew back.

But I was left with a mighty scar reaching clear across my chest and right on into my heart. I was, I was certain, damaged goods. Could I even call myself a "real" woman again? After all, I lived in the United States of America, a breast-obsessed place where a well-defined rack of mammary glands is regularly used to sell us everything from love to fast cars. Society, pop-culture, personal history and a new reality of everyday life taught me that I was different now, and not in a great way.

I decided I needed new teachers.

As a journalist, one way I learn something about myself is to begin by learning a lot about other people.

I went to ABC News and said I wanted to produce a special about five women and how they had gone about surviving breast cancer (so far). Why not share what I was going to learn with millions of others? Why not make as much noise as possible? By 1993, breast cancer already had killed more than twice the number of Americans killed in World War I, World War II, the Korean War, Vietnam and the Gulf War combined. What we had here was an epidemic.

ABC said yes to the show, although we had a bit of a tiff over the title. The media was finally paying attention (although not enough) to AIDS. I wanted to call our program *The Other Epidemic*. An ABC executive insisted viewers were too dumb to know what I meant, to know that the *other* epidemic was AIDS. (This kind of thinking explains a lot about the television you get, but that's a story for another time.) In the end, I won, but only sort of; I had to explain the title at the beginning of the show.

"And now, news for dummies…and other network executives."

Nevertheless, we went to work on the program. We found our women, each remarkable in her way. Sue Miller was one of those women, and from the beginning, it was clear she had something to say to me. I mean me, personally. It was a simple message really, but a fantastically powerful one. What Sue said to me, to all of us, was this: *You do not need to define your femininity or your sexuality by body parts.*

Well, imagine that.

Now, 14 years later, I know exactly what she means. I may have no breasts, and, no, I never went back for reconstruction, but I have my health, I have the love of a terrific fellow, and I have back my sense of self. Look at me. I am girly, womanly, female, feminine, sexy—and powerful. *And I am still here.*

Sue gave me this gift by simply giving me her story. It was during the making of that TV special that I began to see how necessary it was for all of us to tell our stories—on TV, in meeting halls, churches, cafes and one another's living rooms, kitchens (kitchens are special places for sharing stuff) or books. We *are* our stories. More than that, we are women, and women learn from other women's stories, always have, probably always will. Today I go around the country telling my story to as many people who will listen, men as well as women because (A) breast cancer affects everyone who loves (or even knows) the person who actually has it, and (B) men get breast cancer too.

Now I encourage you to read Sue's book. Read it and buy another copy for someone else who needs it. I assure you that any woman, especially one who's just been diagnosed with this disease, is going to profit from hearing the right words, not too many of them and in the right order from a woman who was diagnosed in 1971, and is still strutting her stuff today. And I do mean *strutting*. A "Day of Caring?" Honey, this beautiful woman is a "Life of Caring."

Wait until you see where her journey has taken her. Better yet, turn the page and come along for the ride. I assure you that when you are done you will say, as I do, mentally and regularly: "Hey, Sue! Thanks! I needed that."

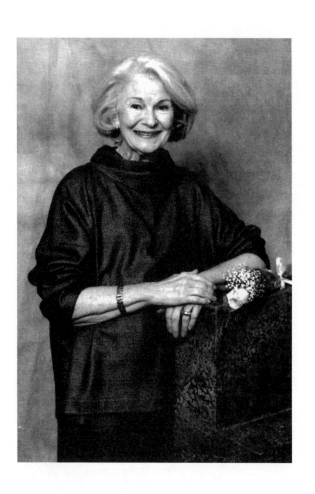

Introduction

Many people have asked, "What motivated you to start the Day of Caring?" As the 25th anniversary of the Day of Caring for Breast Cancer Awareness approached, I felt the time was right to answer that question. To respond honestly, I realized that I would have to tell not just part of my story, but, in fairness to myself and readers, the whole truth.

The Day of Caring stemmed from my life experiences. It pulled together all of the fear, sadness, and low self-esteem I had grappled with most of my life. Because I worked to help other people overcome some of their negative feelings about themselves, I in turn learned how to handle my own recurrent doubts.

On a personal level, I wrote my story to understand it more fully. I wanted to reflect on how I became the person I am today. As I remembered my childhood, marriages, struggles and joys, I saw the shape of a whole life, with definite patterns. The threads of memory helped me see how my life ties together.

I know that as my children read this book, it won't be easy. They will probably think, *Why did she share her very personal stories with the world?* My answer is simple. Every time something bad happened in my life, sharing my stories helped make it better.

Bad things happen to good people, but you don't have to let the bad things color all of the good. Life can be filled with magic if you don't let the disappointments and hurts overshadow the beauty.

A note from Amber

When a modest woman writes her life story, the view may be skewed. She will want to leave out tiny details like how she helped thousands of people. I think I coaxed out the majority of the story. But who knows what else Sue Miller accomplished and forgot to mention; maybe she won the Nobel Prize once and didn't want to make a big deal of it.

During my first meeting with Sue Miller, I saw a gracious and elegant woman. Over our year-long collaboration, I came to know a shy person, blunt in speaking the truth but tentative about sharing it in a book; a courageous person, willing to examine difficult experiences; and a generous person, always ready to help family and friends. I grew to love her.

Everywhere she goes, people open their hearts to her. Her scrapbooks are filled with notes from people saying things like this excerpt: "You are wonderful! You'll never know how much you've given me! Thank you for calling in the hospital, at home—and then for the fashion show."

Sue has enriched so many lives with just a brief contact. I hope this book gives you a fuller sense of her life. The courage that emanates from her slender frame may surprise you. Her spirit will certainly inspire you. Even through the pages of a book, she will reach out and enfold you in love.

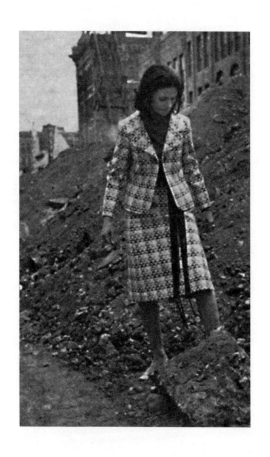

Newspaper shoot when Larimer Square
was in the beginning of renewal in 1971

ON THE EDGE

On a cold February night in 1980, I stood at the top of the Shwayder Theater in Denver, Colorado, gazing below at the metal backs of five hundred empty seats. The stage loomed like a football field at the bottom, decorated with dainty white partitions and a few brave ferns. The emptiness unnerved me. *My Lord in heaven, what have I done? I'll never be able to pull this off.* In half an hour, fifteen women wearing bathing suits, bathrobes and nightgowns would begin modeling "Sue Miller's World of Elegance." Underneath her clothes, each woman bore a mastectomy scar. I set these women up to public scrutiny. Maybe I also set them up for public humiliation.

For me, the show represented a positive response to negative events in my life. I survived growing up with only one breast, childhood incest, ongoing depression, hospitalization after a suicide attempt, and the loss of my job after a mastectomy. With this show, I wanted to do for other breast cancer victims what I couldn't quite seem to do for myself—help them know that they remain whole and complete, still elegant and beautiful.

At the time, people often shunned women who survived cancer and underwent mastectomies. People feared they could catch cancer and figured a woman's life ended if she contracted it. That night I wanted to say to people, "We've had mastectomies, and we're doing OK." I wanted to say to the women who modeled, "Don't hide. Stand up straight and be proud of yourselves." I also didn't want to disappoint my family, who had arrived in force to support me.

Before the show started, I wandered alone through the theater. Whenever I faced something big, I wanted to be by myself. It was easier to stay calm if I didn't have to pretend I was calm. I found talking difficult. My friendships were mainly based on work, which made conversation easy. Until I married my second husband in 1998, I usually kept very quiet in a social situation, afraid I would say something stupid. Looking back today, twenty-five years later, I think it took guts to do what I did that night. I had raised the stakes and waited to see how the evening played out.

As I ambled down the rows of the theater that night in 1980, I heard laughter. I headed toward the source: the dressing rooms. *What's going on in there?* I didn't want to disturb anybody's fun, so I peered around the corner of the doorway. A beige prosthesis flew through the air like a rubber spaceship. "Mine are bigger than yours, so put these on and your dress will fit better," someone called as Adele caught the prosthesis. As I stuck my head a little farther into the room, I saw women adjusting their bra straps, pulling their clothes into place, turning from side to side in the mirror to make sure both bosoms looked the same. Some laughed, others put on makeup or combed each other's hair. They were having a ball!

This differed completely from my modeling career. When you're getting ready for a show as a professional model, you're very serious about how the clothes are looking. You have men wandering in and out, putting jewelry and accessories on you. Your makeup must be exactly right. It's not a fun experience; it's stressful.

Here were women not only inexperienced at modeling but facing a life-threatening disease. Two of them went through divorces after their diagnosis. All of them felt the shock of losing a body part that defined them as women. All of them experienced the censure of a society deeply afraid of cancer.

I heard the bustle in that room. I watched the women helping each other. Clarice, a striking black woman from Jamaica, comforted a short, gray-haired woman. She said, "You're going to walk out on that ramp and shine, darlin'. You're beautiful."

I knew then why I had done all this. Women needed to come together to support each other, to turn a tragic time in their lives into something fun.

It didn't matter if anyone else came. Those women found help, love and support from each other. They were no longer alone. That proved to be one of the biggest realizations in my life. I thought, *I have given these women a sorority, a place to be part of each other, a support system.*

It seemed like somebody put a sign before me that said, "This is what you really wanted to do. You wanted to give them a place where they wouldn't feel like outsiders."

I never did go inside the dressing room, because I didn't want to disturb their time together. When you oversee a big function, you don a certain role. It seemed more important for them to do what they were doing than for them to see me. So I retreated down the hall and walked back to the stage.

For five minutes or so, I absorbed the quiet, pondering how the evening would end. I knew it made no sense to worry; things were beyond my control now. I heard voices from the lobby. I had issued perhaps five hundred invitations, but as a novice planner I neglected to ask for an RSVP. How many people were out there? Ten? A hundred? *What have I done?* Then I started down the steps, wondering and wandering, trying to relax my shaking knees.

By this time the doors were open. I watched people filter in from the lobby. Not ten, not a hundred, but more than five hundred. Soon the theater overflowed with people. They even sat in the aisles. I saw my first husband, Alan, beaming at me, and my very pregnant daughter smiling with her hands folded on her stomach.

I walked to the podium and began. Actually, I have no idea what I said. When I speak in public, I'm so scared that I don't know what I say. It must have been something like, "We are all human beings. Because we have cancer doesn't mean that we're anything less."

As each woman strolled out, I would say how she discovered her cancer and the steps she took from that point: "Kay Enright was diagnosed with Stage II cancer six months ago and had a double mastectomy. She's wearing a LaVida Gordon lounger, a beige dream wrapped in bird of paradise flowers."

Clarice, already taller than everyone else, floated across the stage in two-inch heels and a silk choir robe. Vivian, the woman who appeared so nervous backstage, looked confident and sassy in blue satin pajamas. Lounge dresses, bathrobes, nightgowns, swimsuits … The ladies who wore those clothes had guts, let me tell you. Lined up across the stage at the end of each set, they looked like angels.

When the show ended, everybody in the audience stood and clapped. I beamed at those very brave models. Later, as people congratulated me, I just repeated over and over again, "Thank you." Actually, I would rather have stayed backstage. People complimented me as if I had done this huge thing. I didn't feel like I had accomplished anything that spectacular. Besides, I received my reward when I heard the ladies laughing in the dressing room. So listening to the praise and seeing the tears embarrassed me. I have since come to realize that I've done something very big in my life. I molded my modeling experience and bout with cancer into something that's helped thousands of women. But that night I felt more sheepish than proud.

After arriving home, I didn't think a lot about the show—no big celebration. I just looked forward to the next step. I needed to answer letters, be sure the publicity went to the right hands, and begin planning for next year. I wanted more people to understand that cancer isn't contagious and to see women with mastectomy scars as still beautiful. I thought of two friends who had refused to attend the show because they feared what they would see: a bunch of women who had mastectomies—how could that be fun to watch? *Well, it is fun to watch. And now people know it.*

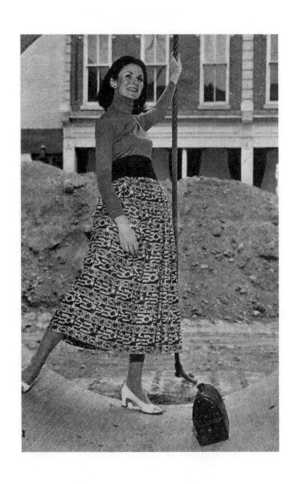

Denver Post *cover picture shown on the Saturday after my mastectomy in 1971*

Overcoming Fear

When surgeons cut away my breast in 1971, people didn't understand cancer the way they do now. They thought you could catch it from a kiss or shaking hands. No one talked about it, especially in public. A diagnosis of breast cancer immediately put you in a state of fear and isolation.

I knew first-hand how hurtful people's reactions could be. When I recovered from surgery enough to resume my daily routine, I saw two friends at the grocery store, standing at the end of an aisle. I waved and pushed my cart toward them, but they turned the corner to avoid talking to me. That hurt.

Equally hard to take was the loss of my career. I had modeled professionally since the age of thirteen, but after my mastectomy, I was fired. Ironically, I had modeled all those years with a "falsie" on the left side. Because an infection as an infant forced doctors to cut into my chest wall and muscles, I never developed a breast on that side. A mastectomy, it seemed, raised far more alarm.

About a year later, my husband Alan took me to a spa in California, where I decided to enjoy the hot tub. I kept a towel on until the last minute, feeling self-conscious. Finally I slipped it off and slid into the hot water—and every woman in that tub stood and walked out. I felt devastated, but I refused to leave. I sat there thinking, *This is stupid. My chest is scarred but it's not catching, for heaven's sake.* Looking at me apparently scared those ladies to death. Granted, I was a sight. On the right I had a long scar rather than a breast, on the left a flat little mass of skin with a nipple, and scars all over my back. Seeing someone in the hot tub looking like that probably wasn't easy for anybody. This happened before any of the presidents' wives discussed their breast cancer, so the public understood little about it. People were very frightened.

It took me seven years after my mastectomy and the loss of my modeling career to muster enough courage to model again. In 1978, on a whim, I stopped at Helene's Boutique, a shop that carried nightwear, sports clothes and swimsuits with pockets for a prosthesis. Helene knew I had modeled professionally, and she asked me to take charge of a fashion show being planned for the Metropolitan Mastectomy Club. Living in self-imposed isolation since my mastectomy, I felt so irritated at the request—terrified, really, of appearing on a runway again—that I uttered an abrupt "no" and on the way out slammed the door so hard it broke. I jumped into the car, furious, and as I started to drive away a light bulb went off in my head. *What would happen if I did the show and used women who had mastectomies?* I returned to apologize, paid for the door, and accepted the invitation. "On one condition," I told her. "The models will be women who have had mastectomies."

A blunt, no-nonsense businesswoman, Helene said: "You will *never* get that done. There is no way anybody who's had cancer and a mastectomy is going to get up there and put a bathing suit on and walk out on a ramp." She finally agreed to let me try. After talking to her customers personally, she gave me a couple of phone numbers. I also approached a friend who held an exercise class for women with mastectomies, and asked for help from women there. After a couple of weeks of pushing, begging and arguing, I found five women willing to participate. They insisted that I couldn't just be a commentator but needed to model, too.

When I walked onto the stage for that small show, my heart beat so hard I thought it must be visible through my low-cut nightgown. When I think about it now, it brings such warm and funny memories. Wearing bathing suits, nightgowns and flimsy little robes is tough when you have nothing to hold them in place. I remember stuffing Kotex pads into our nightgowns so that bra straps would not show. For our strapless bathing suits we taped the tops to prevent them from falling down, but the clear tape kept coming loose. The girls wearing prostheses couldn't figure out how to keep them from falling out the bottom of their outfits. We sweat buckets because we were all so nervous about what we planned to do and prayed we would not ruin the clothes from Helene's. What a scene! But it proved worth it because we had a good time. We forgot our very serious problems in those two hours.

That first show changed lives. One model in her twenties married as a result of participating. She had broken her engagement following her mastectomy, although her fiancé insisted he still wanted to marry her. After appearing on stage in a flowing white nightgown, she realized she could still feel lovely. She decided that a mastectomy wasn't the end of her life and agreed to marry the man who loved her.

Thereafter, I shepherded this small group of women to bridge clubs, schools and other modest venues. With each show I saw their self-confidence rise, and I knew we needed to reach a larger audience. The small shows evolved into a larger one, "Sue Miller's World of Elegance."

I spent months putting together the World of Elegance, with help from friends who liked the idea and wanted to support me. My daughter Leslie said,

"Go over to the Jewish Community Center and see if you can have the Shwayder Theater. It has about four hundred seats and a beautiful stage." I am Jewish and the JCC let me use the space for free. A small shop donated invitations, Sweetness & Co. provided music, and Epicurean Catering agreed to set up an after-show buffet with appetizers and sweets. David Squires decorated the stage. They all did it for free.

I knew that to have any success at all, I would need the help of the press. At the time, Eva Hodges was the formidable society editor of *The Denver Post*. Everyone said, "Be my guest, go ahead and go on down there, but she's tough." I scheduled the appointment and I literally shook on my way down. I practiced my speech over and over in my head.

Although a tiny woman, Eva seemed like a giant eyeing me sternly from her chair. My legs shook so hard that I absolutely needed to sit down. I said, "I have an idea. But in order to make it successful, I have to have the help of the newspaper."

To my amazement, Eva said, "I think your show is a fabulous idea." She gave us a three-page preview in *The Denver Post* Style section. The headline read: "Mirror, mirror: 'You're still a foxy lady.'"

That was indeed the message I hoped the World of Elegance would convey. I thought about how to explain my project in the publicity for the show.

I wrote:

> The World of Elegance is dedicated to changing attitudes toward breast cancer and mastectomies...We first of all tell the woman who has had a mastectomy that she is a woman, a beautiful woman, able to wear basically all of today's fashions. Secondly, by appearing before the whole community, we hope to conquer breast cancer's number one enemy—FEAR. Fear is what prevents a woman from learning about breast self exam and other diagnostic procedures and then following through with a visit to the doctor. Early detection is primary in control and cure of the disease. In our own small way, we hope to ease the stigma attached to breast cancer and to aid in the rehabilitation of mastectomy patients.

I was wound pretty tight the night of the show, wondering if I'd made a huge mistake. When I heard the women in the dressing room, though, everything fell into place. The evening was a resounding success, and in the days following I rode a wave of publicity, doing interviews and making public appearances. For weeks, I appeared on TV, telling my story but also talking about and showing the models.

The night of Sue Miller's World of Elegance, I met Joan Camp, RN, head of the Breast Center at Swedish Hospital in Denver, who gave speeches to small groups about breast self-exam and the medical aspects of cancer. She had seen the show, and we immediately became a team. Joan learned the emotional aspects of breast cancer from my experience, and I learned the medical aspects from her. Joan was truly interested in people. Her smile radiated warmth and understanding. I learned so much from her.

The two of us would visit groups in small towns, one day in Lamar, the next La Junta, the next Merino or Ward. Wherever Joan talked she'd bring me along, and I would give a little spiel about being a model and what had happened to me. As we traveled around Colorado we talked nonstop about how to improve women's lives. One day I said, "Joan, we need to make this bigger. We need to have a day of caring for women."

Joan nodded. She said, "That's the name, Day of Caring."

And from that conversation sprouted a multimillion-dollar forum for education and celebration. I didn't think about the scope of the project or wonder about its effect on my life. I wanted to keep helping other women, taking the next step. A Day of Caring felt just right.

Helping others became my life's mission. Cancer pointed me in a direction I never expected to go. Rabbi Ed Feinstein, a two-time survivor of cancer, says, "No one asks for cancer. No one deserves it. But once it has found its way into our lives, it can become a powerful teacher. Cancer can teach us to take seriously the purposes for which we live ... Cancer can teach us to embrace and celebrate the moments that matter—moments of closeness, of insight, of meaning. We who have survived cancer have much to teach."[1]

Cancer is as frightening a diagnosis as it ever was. What has changed is public understanding. People are more open, more willing to support others. In my own way, I have been part of that evolution. I believe that we cancer patients and survivors need to take our experiences and help other people in need. Our lives are not over. Our lives are better. We have been given a great opportunity to help other human beings see that cancer can become the start of life, not the end.

---

[1] Feinstein, Ed. "New Vision, Wisdom and Clarity." *Coping Magazine*, July/Aug. 2005: 14.

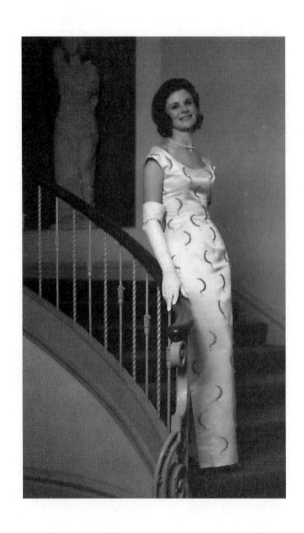

*A fashion show from Duplers furs
at Green Gables Country Club*

MISTS OF CHILDHOOD

The tentacles of childhood twine through our lives, pulling at us even as adults. For me, strands of love, hate, sadness and confusion tangle together. As a scared, meek little girl, I loved my father but couldn't bear to be in the same room with him. As a teenager and young adult, I was plagued by panic attacks. At thirty-two I ended up in a mental hospital, suicidal. All my life I've been unable to sit still, afraid of what might catch me. Even now, at seventy-two, when I think about my childhood, a great sadness threatens to overwhelm me. I have faced my memories as bravely as I could, lived a full and loving life, and even managed to help some other people along the way. But the feelings of my childhood still coil inside me. They are simultaneously part of who I am and what I have overcome.

I would like to pull up the hurt I feel about my father and understand it fully, but I can't. That whole part of my life has a cloudy quality to it. Given my memory of a few scenes and the symptoms I developed later in life, it's obvious that something in my childhood was very, very wrong. My father violated me. Some call it incest, others molestation. But to a little girl, it spelled terror.

My family moved from town to town. I was born in Kansas City, Missouri, in March of 1934. We moved from Kansas City to Boston ... back to Kansas City ... on to Corpus Christi ... then Oklahoma City. I have a picture of myself on a pony in Boston, but no memory to go with it. It's like looking at somebody else. We traveled so much because my father, who possessed a brilliant mind for numbers, was in the forefront of setting up credit lines for large companies. He laid the groundwork for what later became MasterCard and Visa.

I had a large extended family on my mother's side, many of them involved in the family business, a chain of maybe ten jewelry stores across Texas and Oklahoma. My father joined the business with my mother's family because they needed a sharp CPA. The stores held a little of everything—diamonds, gems and expensive costume jewelry. Even as an eight-year-old, I worked in one of the stores, wrapping gifts and doing chores.

My grandmother, Lillian Shoshone, emigrated from Russia. When she arrived in Kansas City, she saw the need for decent housing in the poor areas of town. The bank loaned her money on the strength of her ideas—she signed her name with an X—and she became very successful building apartment houses for poor residents.

My grandfather also emigrated from Russia. He and my grandmother lived with my family the whole time I was growing up. Poppa would sit in his chair just as he had done in the old country, drinking tea with a sugar cube in his mouth and reading the *Jewish Forward*, a Hebrew newspaper. You could be from Russia or Spain or wherever, but the whole world contained your Jewish brothers and sisters and cousins, and you read news of them through the *Forward*.

My grandmother gave birth to seven children in Russia, but only five lived to cross the sea to America. My mother, Tobie, the eighth child, was born in Kansas City. A vibrant woman who loved to talk and laugh, she enjoyed playing cards. There was always a game going on at the house. She lived for her family. She wanted only for everyone to get along. Anger and confrontation frightened her. She did everything she could to keep peace in her family and her extended family, to the point that she gave up many things she loved, like "True Romance Magazine," because her sisters did not approve.

My mother had coal black hair, a ready laugh, and a perennial Marlboro in her hand. Men loved her. If my parents attended a party, my mother always danced. She could never understand why I chose the life I did. Why would I spend so many hours organizing breast cancer events when I could be home playing cards? I remember her saying after I married, "You're never going to have friends unless you learn to play cards." So I did. For a year, I tried to play cards and mahjong, and all I achieved was a year-long headache. Finally, I called my mother and said, "No more cards. I may never have any friends but at least I will not have a headache."

When the Day of Caring began to pick up steam, I would send articles about it to my mother and sister. In 1986, the Day of Caring was under the umbrella of the Nancy Gosselin Foundation, which held a luncheon to honor me as founder of the Day of Caring. My mother and sister attended the celebration. My sister always supported what I was doing but my mother just shook her head in amazement at what I had accomplished.

My father, a thin, bald man, disappeared in the bustle of the household. Everyone would crowd around the dinner table: me, grandmother and grandfather, mother and father, sister Judy, Uncle Mose (my mother's bachelor brother who was always around), and any of the aunts and uncles who happened to be in town. I remember sitting at the dinner table feeling sorry for my father as my mother and relatives talked for hours, discussing politics or world affairs without ever including him. If he offered an opinion, no one paid attention. Eventually my father would walk off by himself. My heart broke for him. At the same time, I felt angry at him because he wouldn't stand up for himself. It was his house and his table. My father seemed to have no place, and he wouldn't claim one for himself.

Later, as a grown woman, I gathered the courage to talk with my sister about our childhood, and Judy affirmed that something was wrong. She felt the same ambivalence I did, although for her it was more a reaction to our father's general behavior and not related to sex.

Judy and I looked like we came from different parents. Judy's dark hair encircled olive skin, while my pitch black hair stood in stark contrast to my porcelain features. Judy resembled my mother, jovial and gregarious. They always played cards and laughed. I was a shy child who never caused trouble; my sister was a spitfire. Somebody once remarked that I was scrawny and Judy said, "Don't ever talk to my sister like that." I couldn't stand up for myself but Judy would stand up for me, even though she was younger. She is the only person besides my children who has always gone to bat for me. As a child, Judy suffered rabbit fever, also known as tularemia, and stayed in the hospital for six days. I never wanted to leave her alone in the hospital. I sat on her bed all day. My parents pried me loose to take me home.

My sister and I are nothing alike, but we have the most wonderful relationship. We respect and accept each just for who we are. We are best friends.

When we lived in Texas, my mother and Judy would go shopping, while my dad would go fishing off the pier in Corpus Christi. He always went by himself, which wrenched my heart. He would ask me to go, but I couldn't bring myself to be alone with him. I felt sick whenever he touched or hugged me. I hated myself for those feelings. I remember that in Oklahoma City he took pills in order to sleep. He always stayed home in bed, and Mother provided excuses about why he couldn't arise or talk to somebody on the phone. I suspected that my mother knew my dad was sick in his mind and touched me inappropriately, but she never could have faced that reality. Although they lived in the same house and discussed their children, my parents didn't have much of a relationship. Maybe that's why whatever happened to me happened—because my father just didn't have a relationship with anybody. He was lonely.

My father felt protective to the point of jealousy over Judy and me. Once, when we were teenagers in Oklahoma City, a bunch of boys came knocking on our bedroom window. My father grabbed a shotgun, ran into the street and yelled, "If you ever come near them, I'll kill you!" We weren't scared at first—it wasn't such a bad deal to have boys knocking on our window. But my mother clearly worried that Dad would really kill them and her reaction alarmed us.

As I grew up, I developed symptoms I didn't understand, including depression and panic attacks. Nightmares interrupted my sleep almost every night. On the evening of my wedding night, at age nineteen and one week, I felt so scared of having intercourse I passed out in the shower. Alan, tender and sweet, knew about the loss of my breast. He also knew something else was wrong because I was unusually ashamed about sex.

For years, I wandered in a world of my own, feelings simmering inside. The panic attacks intensified. I saw doctors who prescribed medication so I could think straight. At thirty-two, a month after my son's bar mitzvah, I took an overdose of sleeping pills to kill myself and was hospitalized for six weeks. Working with a psychiatrist at the hospital, I found the courage to face my childhood and go on.

I always recoiled from physical contact with my father, even with a life and family of my own. He stayed with us when he visited town on business, and I would go berserk. I would wander the house and scream at my children and my husband. My kids used to say, "What's wrong with you? Settle down." Until the day he left, I trembled in terror, thinking that he would touch me or even just hug me.

When he developed emphysema and was dying in the hospital, I flew to sit beside him, along with my mother and Judy. I felt sick the whole time. I thought, *I wish he'd die already.* Then again, I hated myself for feeling that way. For six weeks, each day the doctor would say my father would die. For six weeks, he didn't. Finally I developed a horrible cold and flew home the day before Thanksgiving, only to turn around and go back the next day, when my father really did pass away.

I cannot describe the turmoil I felt carrying those feelings around: to love my father and hate my father, to hate myself, to live in a swirl of blame, guilt, sadness and mystery—no wonder I ended up in a mental hospital. Whatever happened in my childhood has affected my life in deep, irrevocable ways.

But it never destroyed me. Now, as I am in training to be a counselor, I sometimes think, *If I had a patient coming to me like this, I would wonder how they managed to go on.* I don't have a formula for what kept me going. I don't know how I held things together enough to marry. Sometimes I am amazed I have children and could tell my children to honor and enjoy sex with their partners.

I do believe that all people have something in their lives they must overcome. I don't think anybody in this world hasn't come against very hard times. But no matter who you are, you either let it ruin the rest of your life or you somehow overcome it and achieve something with your life. I can't hold onto problems. All I want to do is hold onto successes.

Here is how I deal with my childhood now. I try not to think about it, even though it is always with me. I can talk about it to some degree, being careful to give myself some recovery time afterward. I can list some positives. For instance, I remember my father's love of opera and symphony, and am happy he passed that on to me. I think of his joy at the birth of my son, Bobby. I may have been running through my life, but thankfully I had something to run *with*—my work with breast cancer. I took the negative energy of self-hatred and turned it into something positive. In a way, all my experiences have led me to know intensely what it is to hate yourself, and then learn to love yourself.

The deepest hurt of my life occurred early on. I was wounded as a child. Yet over time I changed myself from a panic-stricken, powerless person into a competent, caring one. I never thought I would be somebody mighty enough to change lives. Yet in my work with breast cancer patients and their families, I know I have done that. I accept all the experiences that have shaped me, because I have become a person who knows how to stand straight. I have looked behind, but my strength lies in looking ahead.

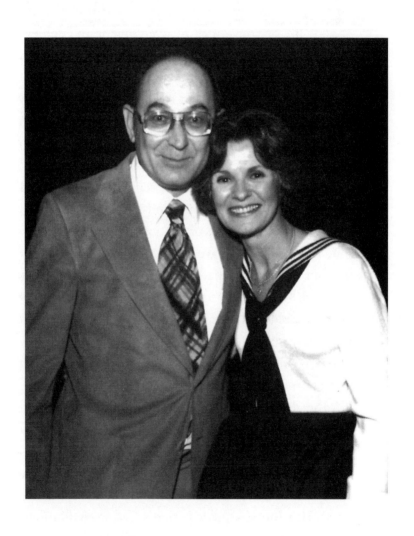

Alan and me at the first Day of Caring

A New Nest

With the impetuosity of a fledging bird, I burst out of my family home, away from the anxiety and shame of my childhood. I fled to the first safe spot I could find, the arms of Alan Stanton Miller, a six-foot-two-inch, lanky cowboy. In his lifetime, he had two loves: me and the ranching business. Sometimes I wasn't sure who came first, me or the cows.

We met in the summer of 1951, when I was seventeen years old and a senior in high school. Alan's lifetime friend Joe, recovering from a recent breakup, asked Alan to go with him to Oklahoma City to visit his cousin, who worked in my family's jewelry store. Alan turned to his father and asked, "Can I go?"

His father replied, "Why do you want to go to Oklahoma City? There is nothing there."

Alan had no sooner hung up the phone than his father reconsidered. "Call Joe back and tell him you can go."

"What changed your mind?" Alan asked.

"I don't know."

I like to think fate stepped in, because otherwise Alan and I might never have met. Alan and Joe cruised into Oklahoma City in Joe's red convertible, ready for fun. Joe had set up a date for Alan with my cousin, but Alan's date and my date both fell sick, so I went out with Alan. I had never heard of a Jewish cowboy before, but there he was, in all his bow-legged glory. We danced the night away at the Black Hotel.

I went home thinking that Alan was a nice man but that I would never see him again. Alan went home and told his mother and father, "I've met the girl I'm going to marry." Being a cowboy, he was a man of few words, so his folks took him seriously. Between that August and the following summer, Alan drove to Oklahoma City to see me every weekend.

In August 1952, I flew to Denver to meet Alan's parents. On the plane I sat next to a woman so sick she couldn't hold her head up or care for her baby. I offered to watch the baby, who promptly threw up on me and later spilled a cup of coffee on my new skirt and blouse. I arrived in Denver stained with coffee and smelling of vomit. I felt embarrassed, but held my head high as I walked off the plane and into the embrace of my prospective in-laws.

Alan's mother said lightly, "You are just as beautiful as Alan said you were," and everyone laughed. Later, as I settled in at the home of Alan's aunt and uncle, Alan's father called. He said, "I can't get to know you while you're staying over there. Let's call your folks and ask them if you can stay here." I didn't expect my folks to say yes, but they acquiesced.

For the next week, I stayed at Alan's house. We toured the zoo, enjoyed dinners out, and took long romantic walks. One night, as I prepared for bed after an exhausting day, Alan poked his head in the door. "Can I come in?" he asked.

"Sure," I replied.

He sat on the bed while we talked. Eventually both of us lay down, murmuring about the day's events, and fell asleep. When Alan's parents came home later and found the two of us together, I felt mortified. I cringed while Alan's parents laughed.

My family was sold on Alan from the beginning. My mother and father hoped I would marry Alan and start a nice Jewish family. My aunt Sonya, a self-made woman ahead of her time, recognized in Alan a kindred businessperson. A successful working woman back in the '30s, she was offered a position at Zales Jewelry a decade later as the buyer for the costume jewelry in all their stores. She never bore children but treated Judy and me as her own kids. She voiced her support right away.

I would laugh when I read Alan's letters. Nearly every day, he would write to me from the ranch or college, things like, "Dear Sue, I rode up the north ridge today...." They weren't exactly love letters, more like business letters, but clearly he was thinking of me. For my part, I felt warm and comfortable in Alan's arms. He gave me a sense of protection. With Alan, I felt nothing could hurt me. He was a tall, strong, quiet cowboy who seemed to adore me.

His family's ranch covered a hundred thousand acres along the Snowy Range in Wyoming, divided into smaller ranches managed by different families. Alan's father had six brothers, and all but two joined the cattle business. They all lived in Denver, buying and selling cattle from an office in the Denver Stockyards. Alan stayed at the ranch every summer from the time he was four.

Over the years, I also visited the ranch many times. We stayed at the main ranch house with the foreman and his wife. It featured two bedrooms downstairs, four upstairs and an old-fashioned coal stove. During one visit in 1952, the year we became engaged, I stayed in one bedroom and Alan in another. Lying in bed, I saw something dark flutter across the ceiling. Then another dark shape flew across the room. *Ohmygod, it's bats!* I ducked out of bed, head low, and sprinted into Alan's room, where I spent the night. We didn't do anything; I just wanted to flee from the bats.

I loved the sense of peace that surrounded Alan at the ranch. I would look at him sitting on his horse with a cigarette hanging out of his mouth, and think, *I'm in love with the Marlboro man.* It was a soft time for the two of us. I never enjoyed small talk, so I felt at ease with the sparse conversation. Everyone rode horses, watched calves being born, spent long days driving cattle, and sat close together without saying much.

After one horseback ride in below-zero weather, I couldn't hop off my horse. I had ruptured a disk in my back, a problem that would hound me the rest of my life. Thereafter, I rode in the truck with the foreman's son to do ranch chores. I helped with branding and giving shots, but shuddered every time the iron sizzled on a cow's hide.

For months after we got engaged, I stewed about how to tell Alan I had only one breast. I realized I had to tell him sooner rather than later. As we sat in the car after an evening out, I said, "Alan, there's something you need to know. It might make the difference between your wanting to marry me or not."

I couldn't see his face well in the dark but I felt so ashamed that I covered my face with my hands. I blurted out, "Alan, I don't have a breast on one side and it's OK if you don't want to marry me." Then I started to leave the car, thinking, *Who wants to get married anyway? I don't really want to get married.*

Alan grabbed my hand, took me by the shoulders, and said, "Well, I have something to tell you, too. I have a heart murmur. So now you don't have to marry me."

His words helped me see that I was not just one big bosom. We both started laughing and didn't speak of it again.

On March 17, 1953, St. Patrick's Day, Alan and I married. We lived in Fort Collins while Alan attended Colorado State University. My father-in-law, Bob, seemed very proud of me. He took me to the stockyards on a regular basis to visit with his friends.

I worked at being a good housewife. I cooked tuna casserole so often that Alan pleaded with me to fix something else. One night I tried to cook a prime rib, but so much grease covered the oven that it caught on fire. Undeterred, I cleaned the oven and invited Alan's family for dinner—even though during our dating days, my future father-in-law had pestered me about keeping a kosher kitchen, threatening to boycott any dinner invitations. Alan's mother, Vera, stuck up for me. She told him, "Bob, you eat in a restaurant, you can eat at her house." Bob would look at Vera with a little grin on his face and shake his head.

I determined to roast a good prime rib. I had seen my own mother prepare it a thousand times and felt sure I could do it. The meat tasted delicious but the potatoes were wretched. I started baking the potatoes in the oven at the same time as the meat, and the insides dissolved, leaving only crusty shells.

Bob and Vera named them Fort Collins potatoes and ate every one.

One evening a couple living next door in student housing came over to watch TV after Alan left to play cards. We sat on the floor, eating popcorn and drinking a huge pitcher of something they called Stingers. *Hey, these are tasty,* I thought, and drank four or five glasses without realizing they contained alcohol. I did not leave the floor until Alan came home after the neighbors left. When I stood, my world began to spin. Alan recognized the symptoms and led me outside to walk around in a blizzard. I felt miserable, trudging around outside wearing no coat while my stomach did somersaults. Finally Alan let me go back inside. I fell into bed, the room still spinning. It was just awful. That is the reason I hate drinking. I don't get happy, I get sick.

Alan graduated summa cum laude from Colorado State University in 1954. Just before graduation, his father passed away very suddenly. I felt that a truly wonderful part of my life died with him. I missed his friendship. Alan felt devastated. After college, he had intended to return full time to the work he loved, but instead was inducted into the Army. A month after receiving his orders to report for duty, I found out I was pregnant. Alan felt angry at the fates that took him away from his dream of working full time at the occupation he loved more than life itself. He never worked with his dad the way he had always dreamt he would, and he could not be with me for the birth of our child.

Alan left for basic training in San Antonio, Texas, while I returned home to my parents. That was tough, and I have blocked out most of the experience. My father treated me with kid gloves then, trying in so many ways to be helpful. But I still did not want to be in the same room with him. Alan drove back and forth from San Antonio to see me whenever he could. The minute I began labor my parents called Alan, and he arrived the next day. I still remember the look on his face, like the baby and I were angels with wings and halos.

We named our son, born on June 28, 1955, in Oklahoma City, after Alan's father, Robert, who also had been born on June 28.

A month later, Alan transferred to Whitehall, Michigan as a medic, and baby Bobby and I accompanied him. We lived in the back of a clothing store, in an apartment with two bedrooms, a living room and kitchen. By the first of September, ice built up on the windows and the sun did not appear until spring. I hung diapers and clothes to dry outside, where they would stay for several days, frozen, like pieces of glass. Eventually they dried, and when I brought them in they smelled like fresh, frosty air.

I remember it as one of the best times of my life. Independent for the first time, my life was my own.

When I had first come to Denver as a newlywed, I didn't know anything about myself. I tried to pick out clothes and could not decide which ones because I feared making a wrong choice. In Michigan, I started to feel free. *You like the pink sweater? Take the pink, then.*

Here I took the first steps into becoming my own person. Whitehall was only about five blocks long, and I walked everywhere with Bobby in his stroller. One day, a hornet landed on his blanket. I thought it would sting him, so I reached in and flicked it away. Such a tiny move, yet I wouldn't have possessed the courage to even swat away a hornet until I lived on my own.

The nightmares that plagued my life for years didn't occur quite so often. For the first time, I felt quiet inside. During the day, I didn't have to please anybody or do anything I didn't want to do. I read, watched TV, played with the baby. If I rocked him for hours, no one cautioned me about spoiling him. If we watched Mickey Mouse Club, no one scolded me. We passed our time in happy activity.

Alan, too, felt at peace in Michigan. He would come home and talk about his day, and after that we would play with Bobby and go to bed. Our whole home life centered around each other and our son. It proved to be the best time we ever enjoyed as a couple.

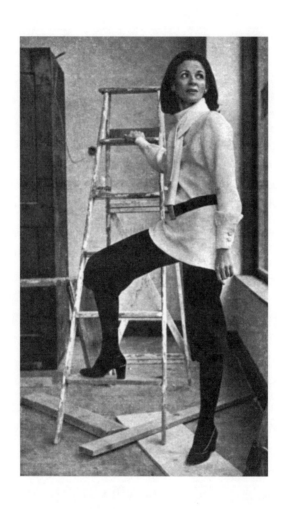

A fashion shoot in Denver in 1965

LIGHT AND SHADOW

We returned to Denver in 1957, three years after we married. Alan set us up in Denver and returned to the ranch on weekends. Our family life changed drastically as our snug family cocoon began to unravel.

Alan longed to live at the ranch, and I was willing, but he also wanted his children to be brought up in the Jewish faith, so we stayed in Denver. We joined Beth Ha Medrosh Hagadol, a conservative synagogue. I never understood the service because it was in Hebrew, but it didn't matter as long as I was with Alan. My views on religion were bound up in memories of my grandfather and grandmother, celebrating high holidays in a little hotel room. Holidays were wonderful as long as the family celebrated together. Today I still believe that being together and sharing our lives is what religion is all about.

Our daughter Leslie was born in Denver in 1958. I wanted a little girl so much. Of course, like all mothers I kept saying, "As long as the baby is healthy, that's all that matters." I feared that if I said I wanted a little girl I would be struck down in some way. It's crazy what we do to ourselves, how hard we make life.

The pregnancy was easy. I loved being pregnant because I felt whole and special. Toward the end, my blood pressure rose dangerously and the doctor decided to induce labor. After I came out of the delivery room, Alan said, "We have a little girl." He told me later that the smile on my face lit up the whole room.

I wanted four children. After Leslie's birth, I kept trying to become pregnant, to no avail. I thought something was wrong and I just couldn't have any more children. Five years later, when I finally became pregnant again, I couldn't have been more thrilled. I used to watch my stomach go up and down when the baby kicked, and laugh. It seemed a miracle to me.

David was born November 16, 1963. In those days, they kept mother and baby in the hospital for a week. On November 22, as I held David in my arms, rubbing my cheek over the soft spot on the top of his head, I suddenly realized the whole hospital was quiet. No one talked, laughed or moved through the corridors. The continual paging for one doctor or another stopped. Even David didn't make a peep. It was eerie.

Then a nurse entered my room and said, in a stunned tone, "Did you hear that President Kennedy was shot?" *Oh, God, no,* I thought. I watched the coverage on TV, and the eerie feeling melted into shock and sadness. I felt sick at losing a president I loved. I remember whispering to David, "What a time for you to be born, little one." He felt so vital to me, a warm bundle of life breathing contentedly while everyone around him seemed immersed in thoughts of death. Several times in my life I learned how precious life is, but David first taught me, when he was six days old.

Unlike in Michigan, when Alan came home for one quiet evening after another, in Denver he was always busy. He routinely played poker and gin rummy with friends, particularly a priest named Father Daley.

One night, when the children were young, I heard a knock on the bedroom door—at 2 a.m.

"Alan, you lay-about! Let's play some cards!" hollered Father Daley.

I shook my head, grimacing. Alan, however, jumped out of bed and dressed. I watched him follow Father Daley, who was swinging a bottle of Scotch, down the hallway. I rose at 6 a.m. or so and found both of them sitting at the table still playing cards. Father Daley had imbibed liberally of the Scotch, although Alan didn't seem to have been drinking. They barely looked up when I entered in my bathrobe.

I hissed at Alan, "I want to tell you something. Your kids are getting up in fifteen minutes, and I want you guys out of here. I don't care where you go, but get out of here!" They both looked at me sheepishly, got up from the table, and left very quietly by the front door. I don't know where they finished their game.

Next to ranching and card-playing, Alan loved baseball. When Bobby was about six, Alan and a neighbor named Keith Starr, along with his friend Alan Hall, decided to build a baseball field in southeast Denver. After they built it, the YMCA took it over, so they constructed another complex at Holly and Yale in Denver, now called the Alan Miller Field. They used their own money as well as donations. We all spent many weekends picking rocks out of the field to make it playable.

For twenty-five years, Alan coached in the Southeast Denver Little League. He became a completely different human when he coached. With his family and with himself, Alan was hard and exacting. As a coach, he was softer. He wasn't thinking about his disappointments in life, or the loss of the ranch, or how his life hadn't worked out. He was fun and supportive.

All the kids loved him. If someone said, "Alan, I need two hundred dollars to go home and see my mother," he would hand over the two hundred dollars. One summer, the league wanted to toss a talented Indian boy out for wearing a braid. Alan talked to the league so the boy could wear his braid and still play. Alan took another kid, a gifted ballplayer on the road to juvenile delinquency, to the ranch with him and kept him there from the time baseball season ended until the start of school. The boy turned his life around, and called Alan regularly thereafter with updates.

My own life centered around home and family. I became president of the Slavens Elementary School PTA. I baked cookies, chaperoned field trips and planned fundraisers. Alan was gone, often at momentous times. When David stole a beautiful coin that another child had brought in for show-and-tell, I took him and the coin back to the teacher. When Bobby threw eggs at a police car and the officers came knocking at the door, I dragged him out from under the bed where he hid with his friends. When Leslie had her appendix out, Alan was at the ranch and I drove her to the hospital alone.

The boys were bar mitzvahed at B.M.H. synagogue and we practiced as conservative Jews. Alan raised his family to adhere to the tenets of the Jewish religion. You don't eat pork, you don't miss the holidays, and you go every day to say prayers when a relative dies.

Alan captained the ship, and his word was law. Only once did I defy one of his decrees. For years I suffered with back pain, eased by swimming. I wanted a little swimming pool in the back yard. "Absolutely not," Alan said every time I broached the subject. Finally, after years of wheedling, I said, "What do you mean, absolutely not? I'm a grown woman. I have a good reason for doing this, and I'm doing it. I don't want to hear any more about it!" I picked up the phone and called a contractor to order the pool—a tiny one, but big enough for me to kick around in and do some exercises. I kept it at ninety degrees and swam every day.

Throughout our marriage, I felt closest to Alan on the high holidays, when he would take his prayer shawl and enfold me in it. In the protective wrap of the tallith, I recaptured the warmth that initially drew me to my husband.

With a group from our synagogue, Alan and I toured Vienna and Budapest. The group decided to visit the World War II concentration camp called Mauthausen, outside Vienna. I flatly refused to go, despite prodding from the group. "How could you miss this experience?" they asked. I knew myself well enough to envision its effect on me. I wouldn't be able to let go of the sadness and it would ruin the entire trip for me. I would have lost the flavor of Budapest and Vienna because my heart would have been so broken by the reality of what had happened in Germany. It's not that I don't think about the Holocaust, because I do. I believe we need to keep that time in history alive so it won't be repeated. I carry those six million Jews in my heart every day. They are part of every Jewish person in the world. I do what I can do as far as helping people and making things better, but on that journey I needed to protect myself.

I spent my time wandering the octagon-shaped streets of Budapest, admiring sculptures, browsing in shops. In my distracted state, I became lost. I didn't

even have a book of matches from the hotel to identify
where I wanted to go. The sun began to set and I grew
scared. I dashed from one shop to another trying to
find someone who could help me.

I ducked into a small bakery and said, "Does any-
body speak English?" No one responded. On a whim
I asked, "Does anybody speak Yiddish?" A gray-
haired man responded in Yiddish, pieced together my
predicament, and took me back to the hotel, which
we discovered just around the corner. I flushed with
embarrassment. I can't quite describe how stupid
I felt. The man, though, just laughed at me with a
twinkle in his eye. "Shalom," he said.

When I returned to my room, Alan said, "Where
in the hell have you been?"

"I got lost," I answered meekly. I feared he was angry
because I hadn't gone to the concentration camp.

"I thought you were never coming back!" he said.
"The room was dark when I walked in. I thought some-
thing terrible happened to you." He wasn't angry with
me for going off on my own; he was simply worried.
The concern in his voice drew the two of us together.
He wrapped me in his arms and we stood, absorbing
each other's presence, grateful to be together again
after an emotional day.

Alan could be so loving. When my confidence
nose-dived, he sometimes coached me about my goals.
For instance, I would receive calls to do print work in

Denver, then worry that I wouldn't be able to find the place. "You'll be OK," Alan would say. "Just go." Each time I located a job on my own, I gained a little more confidence. Once I landed a television spot and felt so nervous I couldn't remember the lines. Alan practiced with me, saying, "No one knows the material better than you. You'll do great!"

He also kept me in clearly defined bounds. He allowed me to model, but only so long as it didn't interfere with family life or his schedule. He withdrew when I needed him to intervene in family matters. I always cowered when it came to Alan's family, especially after my father-in-law died. I always felt a lingering sense of inadequacy. I wanted my husband to stand and say that I was the most important person in the world to him. I wanted him to change his life because of me. That never happened.

I tried to cherish the sweetness there rather than pine for anything more. I appreciated Alan's gentleness and our blossoming family. I tried to outrun life's disappointments and my childhood wounds by staying in constant motion. I wanted to be still, even long enough to enjoy a book, but every time I sat down, anxiety washed over me, a memory from childhood threatening to become clear. I would leap up and dust shelves or review the school budget, anything to distance myself from the looming dread.

Only two things quieted the restlessness. When I held my children, or played or talked with them, the emptiness subsided. Mothering gave me strength to ignore the darkness inside. The other relief came through modeling, when I simply stepped out of myself and into someone confident, without fractures or scars.

As it turned out, though, I couldn't run fast enough, distract myself thoroughly enough, or pretend long enough. The shadows swallowed me anyway.

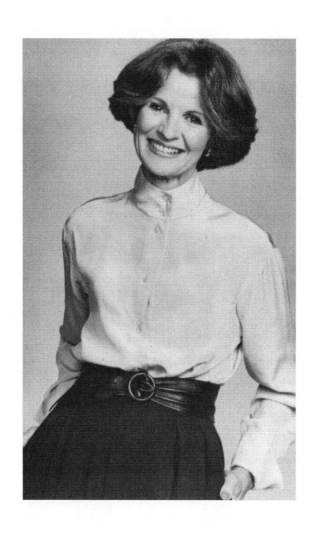

Happy while modeling

Spiraling Out of Control

Everybody endures hard times. Many people have been through far worse than I have. But no matter what happened to someone else, my life still happened to me, and I was floundering.

After I married, I started having panic attacks. One time I hyperventilated in the grocery store and passed out. In the hospital, my doctor said, "Sue, you must see a psychiatrist." I agreed and saw one three or four times, then stopped. That became my pattern. I would have another panic attack, pass out, enter the hospital and see another psychiatrist, never giving myself enough time to really get help. Actually I felt too scared to think about the reasons I needed help.

Panic attacks came when I least expected them. One night Alan and I went to an Irish pub for a dinner party. I walked into the room, saw green walls, and broke into a sweat. *I can't breathe*, I thought, though actually I was panting very fast. I felt like I was choking.

"Alan," I whispered, "something's wrong. Get me out of here."

He turned to me, surprised.

"Something's wrong," I whimpered. "Something's ... "

I awoke on the floor, with Alan's face hovering above me. Anxiety still raced through me. Alan lifted me and walked me outside, where I gulped sweet evening air. After a few minutes, my breathing returned to normal. I looked at Alan and said, "I don't know what that was."

"Do you want to go home?" he asked.

"No, I'm fine. Let's go back in."

He put his arm around me and we returned to the pub. I took another look at those green walls, started choking, and fainted again. When I awoke that time, Alan took me to the car and we drove home in a strained silence. I felt foolish. I had no idea why green walls would affect me so.

Following our son Bob's bar mitzvah, my depression deepened. After everyone left the house in the morning, I huddled on the kitchen floor with my back against a cupboard. I just sat, all day long. I didn't focus on anything. I didn't know why I felt so horribly sad. Thoughts drifted through my mind: *Why am I sitting on the floor?...Why can't I get up and do my work?...Why am I so tired?...Why doesn't someone help me?* Pictures flashed through my head: my mother's mouth, open wide, laughing ... my father's closed face ... the scars outside, the scars inside.

point, I asked to see my rabbi. I said to him, "What's wrong with me? So many bad things have happened. What did I do wrong in my life?"

He answered, "Bad things happen to good people." I expected more insight from him. I don't know what I wanted him to say, but what he did say made no sense. *If he doesn't know, who does? Does anybody have answers?*

As a Freudian psychiatrist, Dr. Mayerson expected me to talk about my past and take control of it. He put me on anti-depressants for a while, to think straight. Later, when I didn't feel so scared, I quit taking them.

As it happened, Bobby's bar mitzvah had indeed been a trigger. You see, the only thing in the world I thought I did really well was raising children. It was the only time I felt happy, contented, and fulfilled. Bobby's bar mitzvah signaled to me that these children would go away and then I would be worthless. I would go back to being the awful person I thought I was, an ugly, insecure woman who could not make a decision. My life would be over without my children.

After I talked about the nightmares I had experienced since childhood, I felt a lifting of the depression. The nightly tears I wept in my sleep began to ease. Although talking about my childhood proved difficult, it felt wonderful to realize I wasn't crazy. The fear, guilt, lack of confidence, and depression began to make sense.

Dr. Mayerson helped me understand the faint-
ing episode in the Irish pub, by connecting it to an
isolation room I had been in as an infant. When I
was born, one of the mothers in the maternity ward
had syphilis. A nurse handled her, then touched me
without first washing her hands, leaving me with a
staphylococcus infection and a scraped chest wall
that never developed a breast. The doctors painted my
open sores with gentian violet but held little hope for
my survival.

"Think about it," Dr. Mayerson told me. "You
were trapped in a green isolation room, separated
from your mother, with all those spooky people in
isolation outfits intruding into your life and body. I
think that experience was a crucial determinant to
your becoming a very private person, and to your
conviction that you would make it, in spite of the
odds against you."

I realized he was right. The doctors had sent me
home to die, weak, oozing pus from the sores of the
infection, and stained purple from the gentian violet.
But I survived. My infection gradually healed. I was
left with scars, a fear of hospitals, and panic attacks in
Irish pubs, but after I made the connection, I stopped
fainting in green rooms.

Dr. Mayerson and I revisited my whole childhood,
particularly my feelings about my father. I vented
my anger about not growing a breast and my shame

about my body. We talked about my marriage … my sense of isolation … Alan's absences … my aversion to sex. Alan had always been understanding about my reluctance to have sex. He never pressed me. After working with Dr. Mayerson, I found the courage to tell Alan why I hated sex. He grew so tender with me then, just held me. He said he had always known that something was wrong. Now he understood. Yet no matter how many times the doctor told me, "Sex is as natural as breathing and eating, it's part of being human," I never felt that way. Intellectually, I understood, but emotionally, I felt too broken.

Toward the end of my stay, I surprised myself by wanting to write a letter to my father. I didn't want to sound angry and bitter; I wanted to help my father. I wrote, "Life doesn't have to be horrible. You don't have to live your life beaten down." He never responded, but I felt better for writing. *I survived*, I told myself. *I can't do anything about my past, but I can dream for the future.* I nourished a tiny hope that my life could still be worthwhile. Maybe in some way I could contribute to the world.

Trying to commit suicide was the most misguided action of my life. I can't imagine what my family would have done. I never knew what Alan told our children about my time in Bethesda, but whatever it was, the children were wonderful. They came many times during my stay and they did not seem afraid.

I told them of changes I was making and how much I appreciated the support they gave me, which I so badly needed.

I remained in Bethesda Mental Hospital for six weeks. A month after I left the hospital, I attended a party at Alan's cousin's house. You will never know how badly I did not want to walk into that room. I had felt shy about being me before, but that couldn't compare with the apprehension I felt as a mental patient. Alan's cousin opened the door, and the look of concern that flashed across her face made me grateful. She welcomed me with a hug, and after that I stepped into the party more at ease. I worried so much that people would be frightened of me. Apparently Alan had talked with everyone about the situation, because they exuded warmth and support.

A few days later, I received a telephone call from Terri, my roommate from Bethesda, who was in jail. Terri needed to see me. So Alan picked me up and took me to jail to see her. Sitting across from me in the visiting room, Terri shook her blond head and said, "Oh, I did it this time. I sold drugs."

I said, "What is *wrong* with you?" I felt angry and worried but I still loved her.

Terri ended up in the penitentiary for a while after that escapade, and over the years she didn't reform much. After she moved to California, I called her one day to say I was coming to Los Angeles to speak to a group of breast cancer survivors. She invited me to stay with her. She was living with a man and his son who both cared deeply for her. I didn't know what to expect. Her place turned out to be on the beach, a kind of commune. At that point I had already started the Day of Caring, and as Terri and her friends all sat around smoking pot, I thought, *This is gonna be great for the Day of Caring: Mrs. Alan Miller picked up on drug charges in a commune.* But really, even that didn't bother me. I thought, *What an experience.* It just seemed so bizarre. I loved every minute of it.

I think if Terri had ever tried, she could have been a successful musician or artist. She painted compositions that appeared almost obscene, dark and black. I didn't want to delve into her consciousness; I just tried to encourage her to do what she did well. But Terri plays her guitar and smokes pot and does the things she likes to do. Now, whenever Terri gets into town, she calls me. I suppose you could call us the odd couple, but whatever it is, the friendship we have given each other through the years is based on deep love and respect. Isn't that what friendship is all about?

Between Terri, my family and Dr. Mayerson, I felt the support I needed to face my life. Dr. Mayerson also helped me laugh again. He gave me a cartoon drawing of a dog sitting underneath a couch. The caption said, "Don't you think it's time you came out from under there?" Gradually, I gained confidence in myself, and began to accept the experiences that had been part of my life.

I talked with Dr. Mayerson on a regular basis for two years, two or three times a week. We met intermittently for many years until he retired in 1999. It was like losing a very dear friend. I miss him terribly. He played a huge role in my getting well.

I felt lucky to go to a psychiatrist and work through my whole life. So many people today can't afford to do something like that. That's why my next goal is to open a free mental health clinic for the indigent and people without insurance, after I obtain my counseling degree. At seventy-one, do you think I'm too old to start one? I don't!

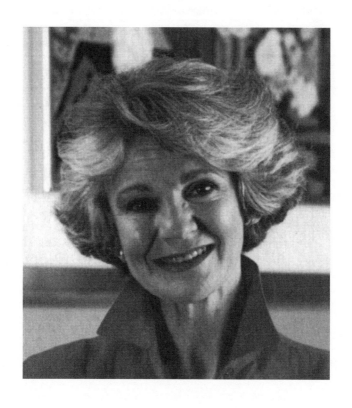

Publicity shot used to advertise the Day of Caring

A Model
with a Mastectomy

Even at six months old I could model. My smile so charmed the photographer taking my baby picture that he asked to use my photos as advertising for his shop. Thus, as an infant, my face appeared in newspaper ads and photography shops in Kansas City.

As a teenager, mortified by my own body, I somehow wandered into a career that emphasized appearance. I became a model at thirteen years old, a shy, scared girl looking for a way to escape her own skin. Some friends of my parents owned a clothing store and wanted a teenager for their television ads. Since my parents could keep an eye on me, they said yes. I did all of the store's advertisements and fashion shows as long as I lived in Oklahoma City.

Right away, I realized I possessed a natural talent for modeling. I had the walk, the smile, the poise, and I never had to go to modeling school to learn how to present myself. In modeling, I seemed to enter someone else's body, someone else's life. Who was this person described by other people as beautiful? Maybe I could become that person.

Shy about telling anyone of the loss of my breast as an infant, I figured out ways to disguise its absence. As a teenager in gym class, I felt embarrassed to see the other girls with their pretty little bosoms. I took care not to reveal my own body, finding private places to change clothes. With a back scarred from the skin grafts and the skin infection, I always faced the wall while changing my clothes, to hide the prosthesis I wore. Most times, I wore a strapless bra so I didn't have to remove it no matter what.

I never complained about the breast loss or the scars except once. I had gone to buy my first bra. I was very small on my right side but it was time to get fitted. For the first time in my life I said something to the lady helping me. I said I hated the way I looked. She looked at me and stopped fitting my bra. She put her hands in front of my face and said, "How would you like to have hands like these?" They were gnarled and crippled from arthritis. I felt like I had committed the biggest sin in the world by complaining. I felt so ashamed of myself. I learned from that experience that I did not have the right to complain. I never did.

When I walked into a room just as me, I always hesitated. No matter how long I took to dress before we left in the evening, I could hear a small voice in my head: *You're ugly. I don't care how dressed up you get, nobody wants to be around you.* I would fret and fuss and delay leaving the house. Alan would say, "You look absolutely gorgeous. What is wrong with you?" As a professional model, though, I could toss my head, take on the role of a beautiful woman, and move with confidence.

A couple of times in my life, I could have gone on to be a high-profile model. At sixteen, I could have modeled for Neiman Marcus in Dallas, which might have led to national exposure. My parents had allowed me to model up to that point, indulging it as a childhood hobby, but when the possibility arrived for modeling as a career, they panicked. That was not an appropriate occupation.

I felt disappointed but I quickly refocused. "All right," I said, "I'll be a nurse then." That sounded even worse, in my parents' opinion: a nice Jewish girl shouldn't be emptying bedpans. I felt my world narrowing again. They wanted me to marry, that's all—so that's what I did.

After Alan and I were married for several years and had returned from college and the Army, I resumed modeling again. Denver offered only limited opportunities, and some of the girls were fiercely competitive. I registered with the John Robert Powers agency, had my publicity shots printed, and regularly checked in at the office, trying to convince the staff to remember to use me. My persistence paid off. One day I happened to be sitting in the office when a model for a bridal show called in sick. The receptionist said to me, "Do you want to do this one?"

You bet I did.

In modeling I detested the "Go-Sees," auditions where clients selected the faces and figures they wanted for a campaign or show. I felt so shy and nervous that I wouldn't talk to the other ladies. My insides would shake, along with my hands if I read a script. Whenever I landed a job, I invariably felt shocked. *Probably no one else would take it*, I said to myself.

During the actual shoot, though, I could mold my body into whatever pose the photographer requested. If the client wanted sexy, or sporty, or glamorous, I knew how to tilt my head or put my chin down or move my eyes a certain way. When the photographer chattered a stream of directions, I plunged in. I could stand on one foot and hold a pose for minutes at a time, while the crew adjusted the lighting. It might take twenty Polaroids to create the perfect lighting for one regular shot. If my makeup began to glisten, then the makeup had to be redone and the shot recast. If someone moved the glass on a table, the shot had to be redone. During all the tinkering, I felt perfectly at ease. I became a confident, gorgeous woman, a woman who could look into the camera with a vibrant smile and prompt anyone looking at the picture to smile back. I loved modeling and could give that love to the camera.

Fashion shows were more difficult than private shoots. The day before a show, the models dropped by for fittings. The next day, they arrived early to have their hair and makeup done. A practice run choreographed the models' movements. All the clothes had to be unzipped or unbuttoned, ready to step into quickly. All the accessories, like nylons and jewelry, needed to be stacked with the clothes. For elaborate clothes like wedding dresses, the models required assistance.

Generally, as the girls changed clothes, tension besieged the back room. "My slip's too long!" a model would say. "Where's the other earring?" someone else would mutter. Voices would cry, "Fix her bra, her pin just broke!" or "I will never be ready!"

A representative from whoever sponsored the show would stand just offstage, looking over the models as they prepared to go out. If the representative approved, she shoved them onto the stage. From the minute the show started until everyone left the stage, panic prevailed. The calmness out front, as models swayed and posed, was a complete illusion.

When I changed clothes, I couldn't do as some of the other models did and toss an outfit on the floor, to be picked up later by a maid. If I wore a five-thousand dollar dress, I hung it up. For one Bill Blass show, I wore blouses that cost a thousand dollars and formal dresses that cost six thousand. I could not throw them on the floor. Of course it forced me to rush more. Including practice, a meal, and the actual show, fashion revues could be very long. Throughout, the models needed to step accurately, descend stairways without looking down, and do everything live—no retakes.

After I removed the clothes and makeup, I became myself again. The smile faded and I reentered my flawed body. My own taste in clothes was simple. My sister Judy possessed the fashion sense of a model and wore exquisite clothes all the time. She helped me pick out an easy, tailored wardrobe perfect for me. Without her, I would never have paid much attention to what I wore. I might easily have wandered around in sweatpants all the time. I didn't buy any of the clothes I modeled, mainly because the discount on the high-end outfits was still outside my budget. *Yeah, ten percent off five thousand. What would Alan say if I bought that?*

When my kids were young, I modeled only three or four times a week. I didn't take on work if it interfered with the children's activities. In 1969 I was asked to be the new Chevrolet girl in print and on TV. I would have to go to New York, work for a week, and come home on weekends, for at least six months to a year. As much as I wanted the opportunity, I decided I couldn't do it. "The most important thing

I do is raising my family," I told my agent. "Find me some more jobs in Denver." So for the next two years I worked three or four times a week doing fashion shows and print work.

In the spring of 1971, I appeared on the cover of *The Denver Post's Empire* magazine for its annual spring fashion issue. As a successful wife, mother, and model, I had it all. Then I felt a lump in my breast while showering. I had experienced benign tumors before, but this new pea-sized knot felt different. I called the doctor the minute I left the bathroom.

I believe the time between finding a tumor and waiting for biopsy results can be the most stressful period in a cancer patient's journey. No matter how well you know that only one out of a hundred tumors is malignant, you are sure this is not true for you. What anyone else says doesn't matter. You pray this isn't cancer; you promise God you'll refrain from thus and such if only it's not malignant. No matter how you try, you can't stop thinking about it. If you are eventually told it is cancer, at least you know what you have to do. When you wait for biopsy results, your whole life hangs in front of your face like some dark question mark.

My biopsy showed a malignant tumor. No one had ever accused me of being stacked, or voluptuous, or even moderately endowed. But the idea of losing my remaining breast sickened me. That little breast provided all of my kids with mother's milk—not fully, but it helped.

"You have a malignant breast tumor," Dr. Cooper told me. "We'll perform a modified radical mastectomy tomorrow morning." His words seemed to hurt him as he spoke. I looked at Alan. The sadness on his face was almost more than I could bear. The doctor continued, "We don't know if the cancer has spread, but we think a radical is indicated, just to be sure." I felt confused, frightened and anxious to keep my family from falling apart. I tried to be optimistic but it just did not work. Part of me turned away from God, feeling picked on, and at the same time I prayed for added strength.

The night before surgery, I lay in bed, my mind boiling with questions. *Am I going to die? What are my chances? Will there be a lot of pain? What will I look like? How could this happen to me?* I needed desperately to share my anxiety with someone, but I could not. I remained frozen in fear.

The next morning I gazed at the anesthesiologist who came to my hospital room to talk. His gray hair and height gave him a stately bearing, but I wasn't reassured. "I am so frightened," I said. "Please help me. I don't want to die."

"Of course we're going to help you," he said gently. "That's why you're here. Now, just relax and take a deep breath."

Next, I heard a female voice saying, "Isn't it a shame. She is so young to have cancer." *Who is that?* I could hear but not speak or move. I opened my eyes and saw the rosy face of a nurse bending over me as she slipped the chart under my pillow, preparing for the ride to my hospital room. I thought I yelled for Alan as I was wheeled into my room. All the way down the hall I thought I called for him, but no, I couldn't have yelled or the nurse would have noticed. I think I felt hysteria and fear. Hearing the nurse say, "It's a shame she's so young," I figured I would die.

How relieved I felt to see Alan when I arrived at my room. As the nurse tucked me into my hospital bed, I focused on Alan's face and fell asleep again.

Physically, I recovered easily. The doctor remained optimistic during his visit. "We got all the malignant cells. Your chances for a complete recovery are excellent." *Thank God. As long as the cancer is gone, the rest of the road will be easy.* With the bandages on, I didn't completely understand what I would look like. On the fifth morning after surgery, the doctor came to remove the drainage tubes, apply a lighter bandage, and help me start doing exercises. "You might want to turn away," he said. "Sometimes women don't like to see themselves in what I call the 'raw' stage."

"It won't bother me," I reassured him. As he cut away the bandages, I laughed and talked with him. After the last piece of gauze fell away, I looked down at myself. I felt dizzy for a moment and couldn't talk. A red scar ran from the middle of my chest all the way under my arm. I looked like a man. *What will Alan say when he sees me like this?* My lips began to tremble. *Everyone will think I'm a man. I'll have to wear high-neck dresses. I'll never wear a bathing suit again.* Oh, how sorry I felt for myself. I hated myself and everyone around me. Yet I forced myself to smile at the doctor and say, "I'm OK." I didn't want anyone to know how disturbed I felt.

I came home from the hospital depressed and sullen. My mind still seethed with uncertainty. Would I need further treatment? How long would it take to heal? Would I be able to swim or play tennis again? Would I ever be beautiful again? I feared I would have no future at all, or one filled only with physical and emotional battles piled on top of my past trauma.

After a few days, I opened up to Alan about all the feelings churning inside me. I wanted to show him what I looked like after the surgery but couldn't muster the courage. I sat on the bed, babbling wildly about this unfair life, my fear of living now, my worries that he would leave me. He said, "Sue, I didn't marry you for your looks. I married you for what is inside you. If I lost a leg or an arm, would you leave me? I love you for what you are." He said exactly what I needed to hear.

In the '70s, people did not talk freely about breasts, much less mastectomies. The word cancer only meant death. Fear ruled the era because nobody understood the disease. Shame engulfed women with mastectomies because bosoms made the woman, and without them, what were you? Nowadays, support groups help women all the way through the process, from diagnosis through reconstructive surgery. But I faced my situation as I always faced difficult times: I shoved the pain deep down inside and focused on something else. I resolved to return to work.

Six weeks after my mastectomy, I visited the modeling agency. Carol, the receptionist, looked surprised to see me. "Sue! How are you?"

"I'm doing great, getting better every day. I want to see what shoots you have coming up, so I can start building my schedule again."

Carol said, "Oh. We didn't think you'd want to model again."

"Of course I do."

Carol hesitated. "But Sue, you know, you having cancer and a mastectomy, well, it's just not going to work."

I shook my head, stunned. "What do you mean? I can still model."

Carol looked down at her fingernails, then said, "It's the other girls. They're afraid of you."

I felt shocked. I considered these women my friends. Not best friends, but people who cared about my welfare. "Oh," I said weakly. They thought I was contagious. I wanted to crumple into a tiny ball on the carpet.

"I'm sorry," Carol said, her voice softening. "They thought it would be hard in the changing rooms, you know, looking at ... " Her voice trailed off.

"Oh," I said again. *I'm no longer beautiful, I'm catching. My life is over.* I left in a rush of shame, hurrying to my car and then the safety of home.

How could they do this to me? I fumed at home. *I am not ugly. I could still model if they'd let me. I wore a prosthesis for twenty-four years and nobody ever knew, so why should it matter now?*

I began dragging out ingredients for a chocolate cake to surprise the kids after school. Furiously I dumped flour and sugar into a bowl, clanging the metal measuring cup against the rim. I spilled cocoa on the counter and swiped at it crossly. Milk, vanilla and eggs. Then I clacked the beaters of the mixer so loudly against the sides of the bowl that my dog started barking and running around in circles. I wanted to take the cake, the dog, and the world and shove them all down the garbage disposal.

But I put the cake in the oven and sat down at the kitchen table, tapping my fingernails. *Fine. I'll go back to school, then.* I called several colleges and ordered course catalogs with a sense of vengeance. Then I pulled out the vacuum and attacked the living room floor, the whine of the machine drowning out any further thoughts of my vanished modeling career.

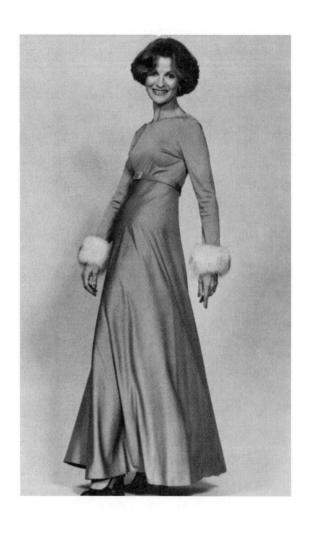

*I was modeling and raising two teenagers
plus a six-year-old boy*

TEENAGE TURBULENCE

My boys seemed to handle the news about my breast cancer without much fuss. Alan talked with them about it in a natural, low-key way. After I returned from the hospital, David came to my room and sat on the bed to talk about his day at kindergarten. He said, "I showed and told that you had a sickness in your bosom and had to take it off." Well, so much for privacy. I wondered what else he talked about during show and tell.

Leslie had a hard time dealing with my breast cancer, mainly because she was a teenager and just beginning to develop breasts, and a neighbor scared her to death early on. The neighbor's child told her that because I had cancer and a mastectomy, Leslie would have the same thing when she grew older. I didn't hear about that conversation until a year after my surgery. At the time, Leslie, certain she would contract cancer, started running wild.

One day officials caught her drinking on the school grounds. They called and I arrived ten minutes later, with smoke fuming from my nose and eyes. I rushed to school so many times because Leslie caused trouble that they named me "Ole Fire in the Eyes" Miller. I began searching Leslie's room regularly, and one day I found a note: "Meet me after school, I have some great dope."

Dread seeped over my shoulders. We always told the children that if we ever caught them with marijuana or anything else illegal, we would be the first to turn them in to the police. Alan was at the ranch, of course, so I would have to do it myself. I thought, *I can't ignore this. I have to do what I said I'd do.* So I called the police, and they were at the house when Leslie arrived home. I also called the parents of the other kids involved, saying, "The police are here, if you want to come over and deal with this." No one showed up.

I thought the police seemed less concerned about Leslie than about me, because I shook and jabbered like a maniac. The next day, the police took Leslie down to the police station, showed her the jail cells, and tried to scare her. After that I kept watch and never saw any more evidence of marijuana. Thankfully, that lesson was all she needed. It scared her brothers so much that they completely avoided that particular problem, at least in high school.

After Leslie confided her fears to me, I took her to many doctors and we spent days at a time talking and making decisions about what she could do to help herself. Because I developed cancer before menopause, Leslie faced a higher risk of getting the disease. Between the doctors, Leslie and myself, we decided that at twenty-five years of age she would have her first mammogram, and starting right away she would learn breast self-examinations and do them monthly. We came through the whole experience in one piece, thanks to the fact that she began talking.

I stayed in charge, despite my internal turmoil. We as parents need to stop thinking we're our kids' friends and be their parents instead. I believe families should have fun together, but a parent needs to say, "No, this is not acceptable, and I'm not giving you a reason why. This is it. This is how I'm going to raise you."

All the kids experienced their teenage moments. One day, when Bobby was thirteen, he and I were at the grocery store. Usually he carried the groceries out to the car, and that day I asked, "Would you take the bag?" He grabbed the paper sack, angry at me. I thought, *Uh-huh. Here we go. It's a teenager here.* I ruminated about the situation on the way home, and then sat Bobby down in the kitchen. "Look," I said, "What just happened is a good example of what happens when kids reach teenagehood. One minute you're going to hate me and one minute you're going to love me. One minute you're not going to want to leave my side, and the next you're not going to want me around. That's very normal and it's OK, and I'll understand." I took a breath, studying my boy's closed face. "Just don't overdo it. Remember I'm your mother and you will treat me with respect."

At one point Leslie and a friend decided to run away and become Mormons. I said, "Fine, I'll pack your bags, because if you're in this house, you're going to believe in Judaism and be a Jew." Alan and I spoke about areas where kids needed to make decisions, so we gave them one place where values stood firm. We abided by the household rules ourselves. We might have a social drink, but we wouldn't come home drunk. Some of our friends at the time smoked pot, which we refused to do.

At sixteen, Leslie visited me in the hospital. This time I was in traction for my ongoing back problem. She said, "Mother, I have this boyfriend, and we may want to sleep together." If I hadn't been tied down to the bed I would have fallen out of it. I thought, *Oh, no. What do I do now?*

I said, "If you're really serious about this, Leslie, then you need to go see my gynecologist, and talk about getting some birth control pills and some condoms, and protect yourself." Leslie nodded, not looking at me. "The main thing is, be sure you're ready for this experience. When you get up in the morning, be sure you can look at yourself in the mirror and be proud of yourself. If you are not sure, then you shouldn't be doing it." Leslie didn't say a word, and I didn't push her. I didn't know until later that Leslie actually took my advice. She visited the doctor, obtained the pills, but never slept with the boy. A year later I found the unopened box of pills in her drawer.

I couldn't enjoy sex myself, but I wanted to make sure my children understood it as a natural part of life. At the same time, I didn't want them to be promiscuous.

As a young man, David suddenly withdrew from contact with me. He slipped into his own world. I kept asking, "What's wrong?" His eyes would fill with tears, but he wouldn't say anything. Finally, after weeks of persistent pounding, he told me he had slept with a girl, a longtime friend, and he couldn't live with himself. He didn't like what he had done. "Oh, David," I said, relieved to know what was upsetting him. "You just weren't ready. When your time comes and you're ready, you'll know it."

I advised both my boys to make sure they satisfied their wife or girlfriend or whoever it was. "You need to think of her first, not just your own desires," I told them.

When Bobby left for college, Alan and I sat on his bed and cried like babies. A few months later, we visited him at United States International University in San Diego. On his desk I saw pictures of me,

Alan, Leslie, David, and the family dog. Surprised, I asked, "Do any of your friends have pictures on their desks?"

Bobby said, "No, but these are the people I love. They're important to me." Bobby, a determined and strong man, always did what he felt was right. You knew that if he made you a promise he would keep it, or if he said something to you it was the truth.

Sometimes that's not so wonderful. When Bobby was a few credits from graduation at Colorado State University, he realized he couldn't make a living as a rancher. The cattle markets had dropped and the family business was being sold. He said, "I'm not going back to school. There's no point. I can't use what I have." He wanted to venture into the world.

Alan replied, "OK, but let me tell you something, Bobby. You're going to have to come home, find yourself a place to live, pay for your rent, and figure out how you're going to make it."

Bobby didn't hesitate. He said, "That's fine."

Sure enough, for the next three years he performed an assortment of jobs that caused Alan and me great anxiety. He called Alan and asked, "Why don't you and Mom come down and see where I'm working?" I didn't know exactly where he worked, only that it was at a bar in a dangerous area of the city. Bobby said, "Call before you come and I'll walk you in from the car."

After we arrived, I looked at my son, startled to see him wearing a band around his head. He said, "Mother, there's a man here who's going to put his arm around you, but don't get scared. I'll tell you why later."

Everyone in the bar wore bands around their heads. Alan and I settled ourselves on two barstools. A large Hispanic man walked over, said, "Hi, sweetie pie," gave me a big hug, and left. Half an hour later, a fight broke out between two men who both pulled out knives. I watched in horror as Bobby jumped between the two men and pried them apart. I thought, *I'm never going to live through this. He'll never live through it. We're going to lose him.* But he straightened it out and resumed bartending.

When Bobby walked us back out to the car, he said, "You see, when that man put his arms around you, it meant that you were under his protection. So nobody would dare bother you." I felt like an actor in a gangster movie.

After bartending, Bobby decided to try real estate. He attended real estate school, passed the realtor exam, sold real estate, and hated it. Then he attended stockbroker school, passed that exam, and hated being a stockbroker. Finally he ended up in the car wholesale business, as a middleman between car lots and rental agencies. Ivy, his wife, came on board as the comptroller. They built the business steadily and now have offices in Denver and Cleveland.

Leslie caused us constant worry, right up until she married. One night, while in college at Colorado State University, she arrived home around 10 p.m. She and her boyfriend, Ray Williams, had driven from Fort Collins to see me, since I had just gotten out of the hospital after being in traction for my back.

Alan fumed that Leslie was driving around that time of night, even though Ray had driven her. He told her, "You need to be back at school where you belong."

"I came to see Mother! What's so wrong with that?"

I heard their voices escalate. While Alan and Leslie yelled at each other in the kitchen, Ray came in to see me. He had a very gentle demeanor that I liked. When Leslie finally came back to see me, Ray turned to her and said, "Your dad has a perfect right to yell at you. Remember he's your father. You have to respect him."

Well, that took the wind out of the argument. I couldn't believe what I heard. I knew right then that Ray was a special man.

After the kids left and Alan cooled down, he walked into the bedroom. I looked at him and said, "Alan, we have a problem."

"What?"

"This is a serious relationship. Leslie's a Jew and Ray's a Gentile. They're going to get married, Alan."

"No, that's never going to happen," he said quickly.

But it did. Ray went through an orthodox conversion, even down to the symbolic circumcision, and married Leslie on July 9, 1978. I was delighted with my new son-in-law, but I still felt like an outsider, proud of my beautiful daughter but not close to her.

As I sat at the reception, eating wedding cake, I thought about my own growing-up years, when I didn't want people telling me what to do. If I hadn't had those two years of independence in Michigan, I might never have grown up. I realized suddenly that I needed to let go. I couldn't say any more, "You should wear a coat, it's cold outside," or "You shouldn't treat Ray that way." I needed to let Leslie be an adult. Today I still believe that is the way to handle your adult married family. I never say anything to them unless I see that they are headed for real trouble. Then I say it once and pray they hear me.

After I backed off, my relationship with Leslie strengthened. Once, Leslie came to the house and started complaining about a problem she had with Ray. Battling my initial instinct to take Leslie's side, the new non-interfering me said, "You need to tell Ray this, not me. I don't want to hear about it. Go talk to your husband." Leslie left, and the two worked out their problems. They built a strong family with their two boys, Jeremy and Nathan.

Ray became a firm source of support for me. We often talked about our goals and dreams for the future. When Ray and Leslie bought a new home, Ray told me, "I'm going to build you a carriage house out back. We want you to know you always have a place to go." He never resented the relationship Leslie and I built.

David, our youngest boy, also gave us his share of worry. When he attended college, he fell in with a wild crowd. He left for college very short of stature, and I suspected he worried about it. He experienced a lot of trouble the first year of school. His grades dropped, so we thought he was drinking and smoking pot.

One day he called and said, "Mother, I've just found a dog wandering around, and he doesn't have any collar and I can't find out who he belongs to. Would you let me move into a little house and keep him?" He had already found a small house with cheap rent.

Alan said, "No, he needs to stay in the dorms."

But I had a sense about this. *This is what David needs.* I convinced Alan to let David move so he could take care of the dog.

David named the dog Zack. He and this shiny Springer spaniel became the best of friends. *See, his whole life is straightening out*, I thought. *I knew I was right.*

When David came home after his first year, he had grown several inches and talked about a girl named Sandy. "She's the prettiest jock you've ever seen, Mother." I could tell from his voice that Sandy would become part of our family. Sure enough, they married and now have two girls, Tara and Alana, and one boy, Zachary, nicknamed Zack after David's beloved spaniel.

During those turbulent teenage years, I felt strangely split. When it came to my family, I was Mother. I could raise the children in the way that Alan and I thought best, staying strong even when things got tough. I loved that role. I felt secure and valuable.

Outside that position, I felt shadowy. My modeling life had been snatched away. I no longer did photo shoots to infuse me with confidence. I only had myself in a scarred body, no longer suicidal but still filled with doubts, stumbling my way through life. I desperately wanted to be useful, to contribute to the world, but I didn't know how.

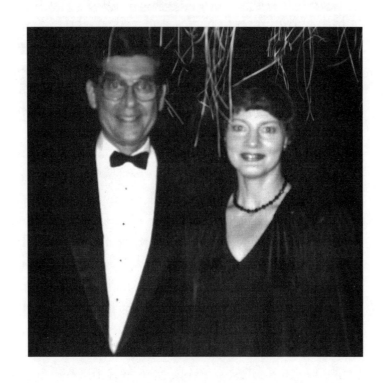

Richard and Joan Camp; Joan was my mentor

Lost Again

After my breast cancer and the loss of my modeling job, I cast about for something meaningful to do. The teenage antics of my children had provided some focus for my energy, but as my children grew older they didn't need me as much.

I had always wanted to be a nurse, and now no one could stop me. I completed a program to be a nurse's aide and worked in a nursing home. When I cared for patients—changing their beds, bathing them, or giving them a hug—the look on their faces made me feel alive. No matter how many bedpans I emptied, I loved nursing. In 1973 I decided to enroll in the R.N. program at Arapahoe Community College.

So many people wanted to be nurses back then that the college instituted a lottery. To be accepted, you needed to be in the room when they called your number. Hopeful applicants arrived the night before and camped in the college gym, waiting for their numbers to be called the next morning. I had a doctor's appointment, so Leslie and Bobby trooped there in my stead. They hauled pillows and blankets, and even after I arrived they wanted to wait with me. We nibbled on M&Ms and peanut butter crackers, huddled together on the floor, and tried to sleep. The room felt cold and crowded, at first abuzz with excitement and then, as the night wore on, tension and fatigue.

I looked around at the crowd of other applicants, all girls in their twenties. I was thirty-five at the time and thought, *What am I doing here? I've lost my mind. How am I going to manage with three kids, if I do get in?* A few girls did a double-take at my graying hair. I kept glancing at the number in my hand: 84. I didn't want to sleep, for fear I would miss hearing the number. *I'll give up cigarettes if I'm accepted. I'll never yell at Bobby again.* Leslie nudged me, reading my mind. She said, "Mother, I know you're going to get in. It's going to be wonderful." I gave her a grateful hug, desperately wanting to believe in a future after cancer.

When, early in the morning, the administrator called over the loudspeaker, "84," the whole room erupted with cheers. My children yelled and clapped, and across the room people joined in. Apparently everyone knew about me, the "old lady" waiting with her kids.

"I'm here! I'm here!" I hollered.

"I know!" the administrator yelled back.

Thrilled, I accepted my lottery slot. I loved everything about the nursing program: hearing about the body and how it worked, learning how to take blood pressure, listening to interesting teachers. There was nothing I *didn't* like. I had wanted to nurse since my teenage years, and now my dream was coming true.

Unfortunately, though, in a sad echo of my modeling career, my nursing career died with a gasp. After graduation, I enthusiastically started working in a hospital. One morning I tried to help a large patient into the bathroom. The patient feared she would lose control, so, with no one in the hall to help, I tried to move the woman by myself. She must have weighed 230 pounds, and I weighed 105. I managed to lurch the patient out of bed, but then she lost her footing and fell on me. It felt like being tackled—a whoosh, a whomp, my breath knocked away, and pain rocketing through my back and legs. We both lay there on the floor, waiting for someone to help. Two other nurses heard the crash of the I.V. stand and came running. They lifted the patient and put her to bed. Shakily, I stood. My back contorted with pain, but I figured it stemmed from old injuries. I had always suffered so much back pain that I discounted what happened.

Actually, I cracked a vertebra, and for the next six weeks, I wore a brace, trying to stabilize my back. I did as much as I could at the hospital, but my doctor told me I would never be able to act as a floor nurse and take care of patients. "You have to quit working," he said. I felt as if the universe sucker-punched me again. How could yet another dream be snatched away so quickly? I was just coming up for my boards, the last step before officially becoming a nurse.

Now, I regret that I didn't yell loud enough. I wish I had said, "I can take my boards and work in a hospital as a charge nurse, as head of my floor." I would have been good at that. But between the breast cancer and the pain in my back, I felt too vulnerable and too tired. I just didn't have the fight. When they said "no," I said OK.

I might have withdrawn completely, sitting in silence on the kitchen floor again—except with my back, it would have been awfully painful sitting. I could have killed myself; once you've attempted suicide, it always seems like an option, offering the powerful allure of a clean ending. The pain would just … stop. But I had already gone down that road and didn't want to take it again. *I'm not going to kill myself over this. I won't do that to my family.* So I wrapped myself in a cloak of busyness, to avoid falling apart. Once again I thought, *I can't dwell on this. I have to move on. This is not so horrible that I can't survive it.* I hobbled along.

I steeled myself to simply muddle through the days. I felt too battered to attempt another dream. In fact, I couldn't even formulate another dream. I kept house and took as much care of the children as they would allow. I learned how to bead flowers, and everyone's houses overflowed with flowers. I listened to music and worked in the garden.

After about six months, a friend asked if I'd be interested in helping her start a foundation for hearing-impaired children. I wrote the first bylaws for what became The LISTEN Foundation and ended up becoming president after a couple of years. The foundation helped hearing-impaired children to listen and speak by providing equipment and therapy. I believed in the work of the organization. I think it nudged me closer to my true life's mission.

The turning point came by accident, when I wandered into Helene's Boutique and she offhandedly asked me to coordinate a fashion show for the Metropolitan Mastectomy Club. I've thought about that moment a lot, with its attendant anger, fear, and, ultimately, hope. I had never expected to model again. Because fate ripped from me the activities I loved most, I had accepted a life where all activities, aside from my family, were interchangeable.

Being fired from modeling had left me feeling kind of crawly. But I think it angered me, too, that people could act that way. Without realizing it, I had been looking for some way to say: "I'm still beautiful and all the other women are still beautiful, and if we didn't have our clothes off you wouldn't know we were any different than other people."

Today, the aversion others showed to me wouldn't happen. Lumpectomies are less noticeable, and the public's knowledge of cancer has vastly increased. But back then, having lost my job, I compressed myself into a tight ball of anger and fumed at the world. The day I decided to do the fashion show for the Metropolitan Mastectomy Club marked my return to wholeness.

Three threads of my life reunited in that shop: breast cancer, modeling, and the desire to be of service. I saw a glimmer of hope, a way to reclaim my self-image. I knew I could help others. Instead of hiding, I could help people honor their fragile human bodies. I could use my experiences to make the world a better place.

I began my new life as an unpaid model and organizer of small shows with mastectomy survivors. As my sense of well-being increased, I began to dream bigger. I white-knuckled my way through Sue Miller's World of Elegance. Then, seeing how desperately people experiencing breast cancer needed support, I planned an event that would ultimately change thousands of lives—the Day of Caring.

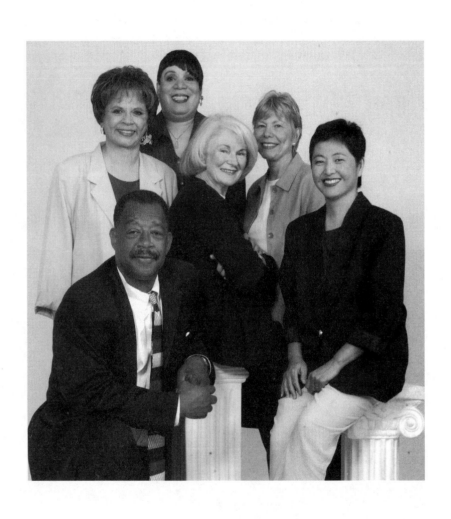

Day of Caring fashion show models
who have all had breast cancer

A Day of Caring

In some ways, breast cancer in the 1970s carried the same stigma as AIDS did when it first appeared. People worried about catching it and shunned those who had it. When I first organized the Day of Caring for Breast Cancer Awareness, people thought you could contract cancer from kissing someone who had it. It sounds ridiculous now, but people really felt that way. Fear kept women from performing breast self-exams or obtaining yearly mammograms. People urgently needed information and support.

I knew I could provide such support. After the success of Sue Miller's World of Elegance, I began planning a similar event for the following year, while still traveling around with my friend Joan Camp, giving talks about breast cancer along with small fashion shows. It didn't take us long to come up with a new name, one that reflected the whole philosophy of our work with breast cancer. The format remained the same, with the fashion show as the event's highlight.

The first Day of Caring, in 1981, took place at the Pinehurst Country Club in Denver, with about a hundred participants. The time was right for education about breast cancer. Because the Day of Caring conveyed a glamorous story about a model who contracted cancer, and because I shared that story with the press, it made the whole concept easier to sell. The media loved this human interest story. People everywhere—at newspapers and TV stations—showed support. I have especially appreciated the ongoing coverage of *The Denver Post, The Rocky Mountain News, Villager,* and *Jewish News.*

The only "education" at the first Day of Caring was that women with mastectomy scars are still beautiful and cancer isn't contagious. More formal educational components grew over time, due largely to Joan Camp's input. Initially the program included addresses by four medical professionals. In 2005, the program featured eighteen educational seminars led by doctors and nurses. Topics ranged from the first year after cancer to the newest information about diagnosis, chemotherapy and plastic surgeries. Over time, seminars included nutrition, yoga, tai chi, and complementary medicine. We geared some toward people five, ten or more years away from diagnosis.

In the beginning, Joan and I did everything: fundraising, publicity, event planning, and coordinating the fashion show. When I ran the fashion show, I located the models, begged them to be part of the event, and met with them all before the show. I became very friendly with them. I loved watching those women, knowing their stories, and seeing their courage as they walked out on the ramp.

I became very close to three models in particular: Clarice, Judy, and Gail. Clarice had developed breast cancer years before, undergone a mastectomy, and never told anybody outside her own family. She was a tall, pitch-black woman from the islands—the only black lady I knew who had breast cancer. I relied on her to model in many shows because no other black woman would touch me or the Day of Caring. Slowly but surely, black women began to come, because they figured if it was OK for Clarice it was OK for them. Underneath, we are really all the same. But it took a lot of guts for Clarice to lead the way.

Judy and Gail had nobody to help them through their experiences. They both suffered alone. After undergoing mastectomies, they ended up divorced. My personal belief is that a man doesn't leave a woman because she's undergone a mastectomy. I believe something must be wrong in the marriage and breast cancer exacerbates the situation. Despite my belief, I felt real sympathy for both Gail and Judy facing breast cancer—and life after it—alone.

Judy, a petite blonde, percolated with anger. The first time I approached her about modeling, she turned away. She felt so angry that no matter what I said, it didn't help. I realized I couldn't do anything for her, so I backed away. A couple of years later, I called again, and Judy seemed more open to starting a new life. After the show she said, "Thank you for making me do this. You drove me crazy, but I'm so glad I did it." I had called her again because I knew somewhere deep inside that if Judy didn't take these steps she never would be happy.

Likewise, Gail felt tremendously angry about having cancer and being divorced. A tall, striking, black-haired woman, she came to my house just after her husband walked out. She completely fell apart as she talked to me. Gradually we picked up the pieces of her life.

When I saw people with potential (and by that I mean they really wanted to get better, no matter what their state of confusion), I pursued them and didn't let up. I knew they would benefit from participating. I knew their self-esteem would return.

Many times I've run into people and known they wouldn't improve. Some people hang on to cancer, so that it becomes an excuse for living a narrower life. I can say to women from now until forever, "Believe in yourself," but one must be willing to take the steps necessary to begin the process. It's hard work.

It took tremendous courage for anyone to waltz onto that stage. I watched many women, no matter how broken, step into a life full of hope. They learned that out of everything bad comes something good. They stayed to share that experience with newly diagnosed women and men.

We did (and still do) treat the models like *Queen for a Day*. They have their hair cut and styled free, thanks to many wonderful hair stylists. They receive a free professional makeover. It's a big party. When you're there, you can feel the warmth and excitement.

For many, the Day of Caring became a touchstone. One girl was dying but wanted to stay in the fashion show. She was later buried in the dress she had modeled, and I spoke at her funeral. After their modeling stints, Gail and Judy started taking part in planning the event. We still visit and go to lunch. Clarice kept in touch until she died in 2004. I felt honored to speak at her funeral, too. Clarice's son, a basketball coach, still calls regularly. I connect with people and the connections don't end. They just keep going on and on and on.

Through the Day of Caring, I saw people begin to take control of their lives. In talking and being with each other, participants formed a support group. They helped each other through the whole process, becoming lifelong friends. I saw women cry together. I saw women with reconstructive surgery proudly walk into the room giggling and then run into the bathroom to observe each other's new bosoms. They shared their lives.

I, too, held a place in the circle. Sometimes I felt like a hostess, chaperoning a big party. Other times I felt like a mother hen. I felt such love and respect for the women who participated. I grieved whenever cancer overtook one of them.

Many friends have passed from my life. Part of me stayed calm and steady as I worked with dying people: Did you prepare your will? Is there anything else you need? What is your pain level? I easily talked with people about dying. But part of me felt completely absorbed in the intense emotions.

One day, after comforting a family, I walked out of the room, bumped into a wall, and smacked my head. I was so wrapped up in the situation that I hadn't even seen the wall. I felt very emotionally involved, more so than I realized. At home, I took care of my family, and the next morning I returned. I might be disoriented after sitting with a dying person, but I could go home and meet my responsibilities, then pick it all up again the next day.

For many years, the Day of Caring *was* me. I put myself on the line with every interview and picture. At one point, a newspaper article showed me looking in a mirror, with my naked back facing the camera. Several people asked, "How could you pose like that?" I tried to prove a point. It seemed like everybody looked at women as though they were only breasts. A woman with a mastectomy was deemed to have no femininity or sexuality left. That picture, though, showed that I was still clearly a woman: pensive, vulnerable, yet graceful.

The Day of Caring gave me the opportunity to use talents I did not realize I possessed. I was a leader who could bring people together and help them find the wonderful resources inside of them to begin a new life. I didn't have to think about it; it was the right thing to do.

It also gave me a certain courage. I had always avoided conflict, but I learned to confront people when necessary. I learned to keep doing television interviews, even though I hated public speaking. My passion about the subject carried me along. I heard myself say things like, "We, as cancer patients, tend to lose a sense of ourselves as possessing a successful tomorrow. We need to remember that our lives extend beyond the anxiety and trauma of the immediate situation. Whatever we were before our surgery—glamorous, outdoorsy, punctual, unorganized, artistic, extroverted, whatever—we will be again when the surgery is over and our incisions have healed. We need to look forward to our future." If, later on, I saw myself in an interview I would think, *Wow, that was wonderful!* Thus the Day of Caring gave me the ability to speak to people and enough confidence to keep going ... and growing.

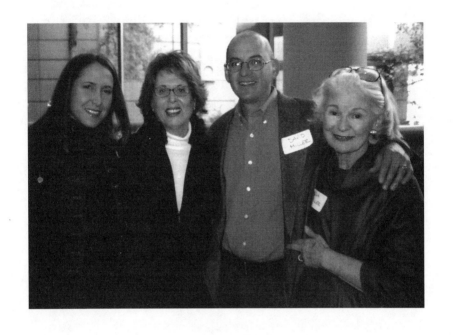

*Participants at Minneapolis Day of Caring,
with son David and me*

Nine Days of Caring

Three aspects mark the growth of the Day of Caring for Breast Cancer Awareness: our first evening fundraiser, the acquisition of a paid executive director, and our expansion into cities nationwide.

As the Day of Caring grew, we remained committed to our primary goal. We refused to turn it into a place where pharmaceutical companies could sell drugs, or doctors could talk about esoteric interests. The focus has always been on cancer patients and their families. The program tries to fill *their* needs.

Initially, women needed to be reassured that they were still beautiful. They still need that, but now people need more. They want information about choices, how to be a full partner in a medical team, and how to advocate with employers, insurance companies and doctors. They want a copy of our resource book, so we give away 25,000 copies in Spanish and English. Some women need scholarships, so we provide up to four hundred a year.

One might think that with its national exposure and recognized quality, the Day of Caring would be home free. But like many nonprofit organizations, it has always lived a precarious existence, with its planners scrambling year-round for funding. In general, the Day of Caring struggles every year. The audio-visual equipment alone costs a fortune now because every doctor wants a screen and spotters and equipment.

At first, I covered expenses with my own money, supplemented by ticket sales. Then Joan and I found small support from a few different sources. Early sponsors included Swedish Medical Center and Hyde Park Jewelers, and later, Foley's and Cherry Creek stores. As the event blossomed, we sought more sponsors. No single source covers our budget. Different sponsors cover different parts (luncheon, seminars, publicity, tapes) for $5,000 or $10,000 each. We have never seen a profit, just covered expenses.

Somehow it's harder to raise money when it's not for research. It's surprisingly difficult to convince people that education is worthwhile. The constant search for funding has been the only discouraging aspect of the Day of Caring for me. When I know I don't have enough money and have to figure out how to keep going without cutting something, I panic. I still make phone calls, I still talk to people about it. The Day of Caring Board does fundraising, and board members work very hard to make the Day of Caring what it is. Finances are a worry for them, too.

I wish a wealthy philanthropist would recognize the importance of the Day of Caring in helping to improve the lives of men and women with breast cancer. Now, even people who don't have breast cancer come to learn. We see 1,000 to 1,200 breast cancer survivors every year. Long-term financial support from a big sponsor would be a relief.

Three supporters in particular have helped ease this burden. One of my longtime allies has been Steve Rosdal with Hyde Park Jewelers. He and Michael Pollack believed in the idea and wanted to contribute. Steve came to me and said, "I want to do a fundraiser for the Day of Caring." He envisioned an Evening of Caring, which took place on April 30, 1988. I co-chaired the event with Steve and my daughter Leslie.

The theme for the Evening of Caring, held at the Tamarac Square Mall, was "Swan Lake." We decorated tables with rose cloths and swan centerpieces. Slipcovers resembling pink satin hearts adorned the chairs. Billowing lace banners hung from the ceiling. On the stage, a huge blue swan swam in an ocean of white cloth. Even the invitations for the event, white swans on a lily pond dotted with rhinestones, received notice in "The Year's Best" list of society columnist Joanne Davidson.

The evening consisted of cocktails, dinner, a silent auction, and what had become my trademark: a fashion show. Tamarac Square provided the clothing, one formal and one casual set for each model. In closing the event, Steve presented me with a check for $10,000 from the Tamarac Square merchants. In all, the event raised around $32,000 for the Day of Caring. That was the first time I ever raised any substantial money.

At that first Evening of Caring, a man with blond hair and a smiling face approached me. Larry Mizel was recognizable at many social events and gave money to numerous organizations. He also believed in what I was doing, and has given money to the Day of Caring every year since. He has always been there, no matter what I've wanted to do. It's been wonderful. I am forever grateful to Larry. I don't think he even realizes the tremendous good he does in this community. He's a man with a big heart.

We held a second Evening of Caring in 1990, raising even more money. Tamarac Square tented the whole outdoor parking area and decorated it like *Alice in Wonderland*. Because the Day of Caring itself grew at such a fast pace, we held only two Evenings of Caring.

I always believed that the Day of Caring should be community-based, not affiliated with any particular university or hospital. The community would give the day its depth and strength. I was, however, a practical woman, and I knew an organizational sponsor would help. The Breast Center at Swedish Hospital initially hosted the Day of Caring. The center allowed us to use its name on the literature; Joan and I did the work and supplied the money. I always retained ownership of the idea. I controlled whether or not the event happened.

In 1987, the Nancy Gosselin Foundation agreed to sponsor the Day of Caring. In 1992, the AMC Cancer Research Center took over the programs of the Nancy Gosselin Foundation. I retained all rights to the Day of Caring, but AMC agreed to be the presenting sponsor. Originally a tuberculosis treatment center, AMC shifted its identity to a cancer treatment center, then a cancer research center. Its mission changed, but community support continued. It became one of the first organizations in the country to focus on cancer treatment and prevention.

I joined the AMC Board of Directors in 1993, volunteering all my time. In 1995, when I had no health insurance and needed a job with benefits, AMC took me on as a paid staff member. I worked at learning how to use a computer and make the Day of Caring more professional. AMC also authorized a team of staff members to help organize the event.

In a stroke of good fortune, Elise Spain chose to work with the Day of Caring team. Her mother died of ovarian cancer when Elise was eight. When she turned forty-three, the same age her mother was when she died, Elise decided to leave her business career and focus on a cause she really believed in. She wanted more than a job; she wanted to pursue a passion and actually make a difference in people's lives.

We began collaborating and formed a mutual fan club. I think that Elise cares as much for the welfare of people as I do. It's like our hearts are twins. She could command three times the salary we pay her, but I know her spirit is with the Day of Caring. For her part, Elise told me once, "Sue, you're the most democratic person I've ever met. Instead of drawing a circle that excludes anybody, you draw the circle around everyone." Actually, we worked together to enlarge the Day of Caring circle.

Gradually Elise took over the day-to-day planning. In 1998, she became the national director to manage the Denver event and develop sites in other cities. Elise gave the Day of Caring the professionalism it needed. She made it bigger and better.

Over the years we outgrew our venues, moving from the country club to hotels to our current location, the cavernous Merchandise Mart. Unbelievably, we manage to fill the space. Between workshops, massage rooms, lectures, a silent auction, gift table, educational booths, and of course the luncheon and fashion show, the place hums with activity and conversation. The year 1998 marked the first time men participated as models in the show, with the appearance of two Denver businessmen. The 24th Day of Caring drew 1,200 people, twelve times its original number. That growth has amazed me, even though I continue to contribute to the growth by speaking on television and giving interviews.

The Day of Caring began to branch out from Denver—first to Hays, Kansas, after a visit Joan and I made in 1981. We gave a talk at the hospital. The coordinators loved the idea of the Day of Caring. Using the Denver day as their blueprint, they started an event that is still going on. People from surrounding farms and ranches model; local nurses and doctors give the seminars. Their site draws 150 people, which is huge for their area. It brings home all that the Day of Caring encompasses: love, education and affirmation.

After AMC Cancer Research took the Day of Caring under its umbrella, new sites opened all over the United States, facilitated by AMC's organizational structure. With nine different Days of Caring, Elise and I traveled to every city. We participated in golf tournaments providing proceeds from their silent auctions to the Day of Caring. We organized auctions and spoke at luncheons. Elise and I met each other coming and going.

It took a huge amount of work to coordinate all those cities and golf tournaments. In order for Elise to focus on Denver, we needed somebody to take over the national Day of Caring. Unfortunately, we couldn't raise the money—it would have taken $50,000 to pay a national director—so we decided to let the other sites continue on their own.

In taking the Day of Caring name, they agreed to follow the pattern we set of education and a fashion show incorporating models with mastectomies. We prohibited them from making the day a fundraiser. It was an educational program, period.

I have visited all of the Day of Caring sites: St. Louis; Baltimore; Palm Springs; Miami; Chicago; Minneapolis; Riverside, California; and Hays, Kansas. Every one contains its own little nucleus, but they're all similar. Some have gotten bigger, and one folded, but Elise and I still feel we reached the right decision. We couldn't kill ourselves trying to ensure that multiple sites worked. We concentrated on making the Denver Day of Caring the best model it could be.

I never expected this tiny fashion show to become a national event. I never sensed that the Day of Caring would become as big as it has. I always thought of it as small seminars sponsored as a temporary venture and I prayed there would be no need for it in the very near future. I hoped cancer would be cured and we wouldn't have to worry about continuing. Instead, the demand is greater than ever. As long as there is a need for the Day of Caring it will be there, with or without me.

Looking over twenty-four years of the event, I almost can't believe it. I attended the Day of Caring in 2005 and thought, in a moment of self-congratulation, *Look what you've done.* People kept saying, "Thank you for starting this." I thought to myself, *Look, you actually are like those people you read about, who do something that changes lives.* I had read many articles in magazines about people who started organizations and projects, and that day I realized that I was one of them. The thought absolutely amazed me. Although Joan and Elise encouraged me and made the Day of Caring bigger and better, basically it was my idea, born of my anger and disappointment.

By all accounts—attendance, longevity and reviews—we're doing a good job. A typical evaluation will say, "Thank you for being there for me when I needed exactly what the Day of Caring was able to provide. I'm so grateful that you were there when I needed it the most." Someone else will write, "It's a wonderful experience to be with others who are fighting the same battle," or "This is such an encouragement for breast cancer survivors and their support people." Participants truly are grateful, and it warms my heart that the Day of Caring fulfills a genuine need.

Building the Day of Caring lifted my self-esteem, helping me to believe in myself. It brought out the best in me, strengthening the parts I most honored.

It showed people watching me, especially my family, that when bad things happen you can take hold of your life again.

I put my whole self into it. Even when I began to feel overwhelmed with the time it took, I needed to keep going. After all, I taught other people not to give up.

I do realize the impact of my work on people's lives. Everybody wants to change the world in some way. We want to leave something important after we are gone. I've done that. I've helped change the way people felt about their lives. Some people walk into the Day of Caring, then walk out, and their life is better, either through a seminar or meeting a friend or seeing the show. I think with some awe about the thousands and thousands of men and women who have passed through my life and how each and every one of them gave me their special gift, the joy of seeing them stride into the future.

I wonder if I was destined to create the Day of Caring. Body image surrounded so much of my life. Maybe God said, "OK, she's a couple of days old and she's not to have a breast. That'll move her in the right direction." Or maybe chance brought that around. When the Pandora's box of my life opened, surprises and stings poured forth. Rather than closing the lid, I followed disappointment where it led. I followed it through abuse and breast cancer.

Eventually I learned to value my experiences. I accepted my pain, looked for the good in it, and wrapped the lessons into the Day of Caring.

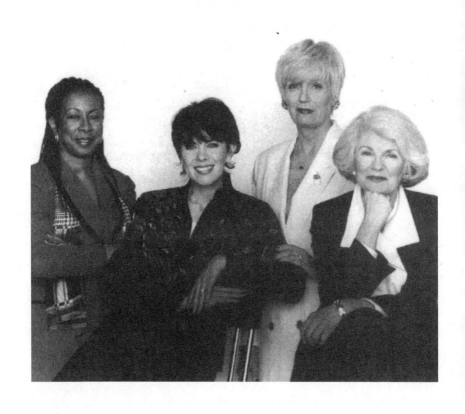

Some of the beautiful past chairwomen of Day of Caring

Embracing Opportunities

I saw the Day of Caring begin a healing process for so many women. I didn't realize until writing this book that I was also trying to heal myself. I wanted women to see their beauty, even though I didn't see my own. I wanted society to accept women with breast cancer, even though I hid myself for so many years. The Day of Caring changed me. The messages I kept giving to everyone else finally sank into my own mind. As a result, I became much happier and more active.

I began paid modeling again in 1983. My friend Jo Farrell, who headed JF images, saw publicity about the Day of Caring and put me back to work as a professional model doing shows for malls, trade shows and print ad campaigns.

Jo protected her models, particularly me. At one shoot, booked as robes and nightgowns, I found an array of lingerie in the changing room. Dismayed, I called Jo. "Look," I said. "Modeling robes is one thing, but I'm not doing bras and panties and girdles. I'm a married woman!"

"What are you talking about?" Jo asked in surprise. Half an hour later, she came flying into the room and started hollering at the man who booked the shoot, while the models stood in the corner and watched. Her voice boomed through the room.

"Don't murder him!" I called out, watching the scene. We all stormed out following Jo, our fiery protector, without modeling any lacy brassieres.

I did many covers for the *The Denver Post* as a regular in the seasonal fashions section. I adorned the cover of *Empire* magazine and other Colorado publications. I did ads for many restaurants, Sears, Frontier Airlines and 7-Up. Whenever I saw myself on a cover, I felt a jolt of surprise. *Who is that woman? Is it possible I'm that pretty?* I felt so unattractive as I struggled through life.

My reconciliation with my glamorous self came gradually. In a profession that prizes youthful appearance, I actually became more at ease with age. When I was fifty, modeling coats at the luxurious Broadmoor Hotel in Colorado Springs, I not only spent the shoot feeling beautiful, but for two days I felt like the most incredible person in the world. After working all day, I ate dinner in a gorgeous dining room at the hotel. I walked into the room without feeling self-conscious about being alone. I knew I looked beautiful, and I stood tall and almost regal. That's the way I felt.

Looking at the menu, everything sounded delectable. I ordered prime rib, a twice-baked potato and Caesar salad. For dessert I asked for a chocolate soufflé drenched in vanilla crème sauce, something I knew I should never eat. That night I suffered a stomach ache and diarrhea. As I slumped on the bathroom floor, I thought, *That's what you get for thinking you're so great.*

The modeling job I most enjoyed took place in Cancun. I was hired, along with four younger people and an older man, to do a resort brochure in Playa del Carmen, Mexico. For two weeks, we rose at 5 in the morning, applied our makeup and spent the whole day shooting on the beach among the Mayan ruins. I was paired with the older man, who sulked because he wanted to be shown with a younger babe. I laughed at that. Though I sported gray hair, my smile sparkled. It was the best-paying and most-fun assignment I ever had.

My paid modeling career spanned fifty years. My face is still in newspapers and magazines as coverage of the Day of Caring becomes better and bigger. I appeared on my last cover, the April 20, 1995 "Spotlight" section of *The Denver Post*, at sixty-two, white-haired, glittering with pearls and swirling the skirt of a lilac gown. "Feeling good, Looking good," the headline read.

Unlike many headlines from my earlier years, this one reflected truth. As a young, vulnerable woman, with each modeling assignment I stepped out of myself and into someone else. As I grew older, modeling nudged me to integrate the picture of myself with my inner self. Gradually, I reconciled the person smiling on the cover with the person smiling inside. Yes, I can say now, with happy surprise: That's me.

I also embraced a more public life when I participated in a special for ABC television called, "The Other Epidemic." It highlighted three different women and how they handled breast cancer. A woman I worked with when she had breast cancer knew journalist Linda Ellerbee and gave her a newspaper story about me that had appeared in *The Denver Post* in 1986. It fit right into Ellerbee's project, and she called me. I don't remember what I said, I was in such a state of shock.

Linda sent a camera crew to follow me around for a week—watching me work with patients and plan the Day of Caring. They also interviewed Alan and the children and recorded a fashion show at Tamarac Square. For that week, I lived with a microphone attached to me twelve hours a day and several crew members hovering everywhere I went. It felt exciting—and exhausting.

The night the special aired on television, I was a nervous wreck. It's uncomfortable to watch yourself, your husband, and your children aired on TV in such a personal way. I sat there in wonder. I wanted to watch and at the same time felt embarrassed. I never moved from my seat until it ended. I watched the special many times before I could comprehend the full meaning. This really meant the big time, appearing on prime time television to share my message with others. We had come a long way, me and all the people who accompanied me on my journey. You may have a good idea, but it takes a lot of people to believe in you and your idea.

My face appeared everywhere, it seemed. Because of my increasing name recognition, in 1992 the state Republican committee asked me to run for the House of Representatives. I lived in a swing district that could determine the political majority in the state House. The GOP was prepared to pour money into the race. I had been a Democrat my entire life, but I thought it sounded fun to enter politics, so I switched parties to run. I also wanted to voice my opinions about certain matters, which, if heard by the Republican committee members, might have given them second thoughts about recruiting me.

Before I ran for office, I insisted on working for my friend, Senator Dottie Wham. Dottie introduced me to legislative life and networking as I worked for a year as one of her assistants. I learned a lot about political life. Then Dottie found me a campaign manager and we set to work. I never expected to win, never in a hundred years. But if I could persuade people to listen to me, it would be worth it.

My platform consisted of education (strong basic education and community involvement), health care (affordability), crime and youth violence (prevention and stiff penalties), and the economy (free enterprise). Mainly, though, I wanted to talk about abortion and homelessness. Some Republicans do believe in abortion, and I'm one. It's none of your business and none of my business to tell anyone what to do with her body; it's each human being's decision. I also said the government shouldn't run the country. The Republicans cut welfare money so homeless people lived on the street without any resources to survive or change their lives. I wanted government programs for schools to stop being cut. I wanted a national health care system. Actually, I was speaking mostly Democrat!

My opponent Ken Gordon and I enjoyed a surprisingly cordial race, perhaps because our beliefs didn't differ dramatically. Ken agreed to have dinner with me. Afterward, he said I reminded him of his mother, and that if I ran in another district he would think it was great.

The Denver Post endorsed my candidacy, saying, "Miller has a fine record of volunteer activities and has been especially active in the crusade against breast cancer. Miller has the kind of rare human qualities that bring out the best in people and would be a breath of fresh air in the Statehouse."

I looked at the process as a game. If I won, fine and dandy. If I didn't, at least I had voiced my opinions. I worked my butt off, let me tell you, trying to be everything to everybody. But it was fun as well. I met all these different people. Win, lose, or draw, I loved the experience.

It was daunting to go door to door talking with voters. I always had a companion, either one of my kids or someone from my election committee. I lost seven pounds walking through neighborhoods all the time. Some nasty people turned me away roughly. Some wouldn't come to the door at all, though I could see them peeking around the curtains. And some wouldn't let me go, corralling me for half an hour talking about politics. Sometimes I met people who made a lot of sense. It surprised me, though, that here I was, a person running for a government office so I could help people, and they could be so nasty. Some wouldn't even listen to another side. That's the problem with politics.

When it came time to vote, I received 40 percent, a huge draw for a newcomer. The Republican committee said, "In two years, you're in for sure."

I said, "No way in hell would I do this again."

I was tired of the nastiness I experienced. A member of my campaign staff encouraged me to put my opponent in a very bad light, but I couldn't do it. Toward the end of the race, unbeknownst to me, the staffer put out a negative flier about what Ken Gordon had said and done. Someone said to me, "We were going to vote for you until you did that."

I replied, "I didn't even know this was coming out."

But of course it was too late.

After the election I switched my party affiliation back and thought about running against Gordon as a Democrat. But I changed my mind again. No matter which party I ran under, I didn't like the compromises inherent in politics. You had to promise so many people so many things that you couldn't perform the job you needed to do. I didn't want to worry about winning next year; I wanted to get in there and do something. It just wasn't for me.

I look back at that time with fondness. I was busy, of course, but emotionally I felt strong and happy. Just as you think that life has finally stopped changing and you're on an even keel, it shifts again. Some changes are good, some bad, but there are you again, adjusting.

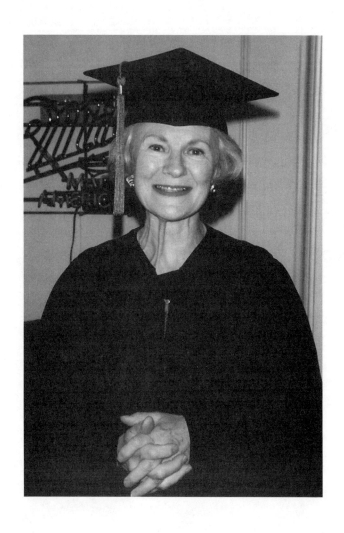

My graduation from college, 1995

SORROW KNOCKS

After Alan's family sold the ranch in Wyoming, Alan's health began deteriorating. The last remnant of his childhood dream disappeared, and I watched as my husband gradually lost the will to live.

Alan was petrified of doctors. Several years before his death in 1995, he fainted on the baseball field. At the hospital, his blood pressure spiked so high it seemed he might explode. I told the nurse, "You take that I.V. out of his hand and the oxygen out of his nose, and he'll be fine." I was right. As soon as they detached the equipment, his blood pressure returned to a safe level.

The doctor told Alan, "You need to stop smoking, and we need to do some tests because something is wrong." Alan needed to hear no more. He never returned. He had a serious ailment, probably clogged arteries, but nobody identified it because he wouldn't be tested. I knew he had great difficulty walking, sitting down after three or four steps. He sweated profusely and began to lose weight. I talked to him about it, but I couldn't convince him to see the doctor.

I anticipated Alan's death for a year before it hap-
pened. I woke in the middle of the night to find him
hanging over the side of the bed, unable to breathe.
"Let's go to the hospital," I said. He refused.

After a baseball tournament one weekend in July
1995, he arrived home too tired to talk. His mother
and all of our children came to our house for dinner,
an unusual occurrence for a Monday. After dinner,
everyone left early. I slipped into bed beside Alan and
kissed him goodnight. Ten minutes later he was dead.
He had experienced a massive coronary. *It finally
happened,* I thought. It wasn't a deep shock to me. I
called 911, opened the front door, and came back and
sat with Alan.

All the children and grandchildren, along with
Alan's mother and my sister and brother-in-law, ar-
rived to sit shiva, a week-long period of mourning.
The kids felt angry. They loved their father a great
deal, and he had left them. They felt upset because he
refused to see a doctor, even though he knew he was
sick. Everyone was on edge and apt to cry at anything.
Someone suffered hurt feelings when I wanted soup
instead of salad for dinner.

I became so stressed that I thought I was having
a heart attack myself. I left for the hospital, asking
Bobby to drive me, without telling anyone else. Of
course when the other kids found out, they were furi-
ous. "How could you take Mom to the hospital with-

out saying anything?" they shouted at Bobby. They feared I would die, too. I was OK, though— just suffering from plain old stress.

That week of shiva ended with everyone yelling at everyone else. Finally I said to my children and their spouses, "Tomorrow night I want all six of you of here for dinner. No grandkids, no dogs, just you and me." When we all sat down together the next night, I looked at their anxious faces and said, "Your daddy is dead. There is nothing we can do about it. I know you're all angry and upset, but we're taking this anger out on each other. Do we want to lose each other, too? Let's stop doing that."

The anger and fear came pouring out then, as everyone talked and cried. Tears flowed freely, but at the end of the evening our hearts lifted a little. It was the beginning of healing.

Ordinarily in the Jewish religion, the deceased's relatives will visit the synagogue to pray twice a day for a year. The kids asked if I wanted them to do that. "It's up to you," I told them. "You do what you want to do. You gave him everything you had to give, while he was alive. He's dead, so he's not going to know the difference now. It's what you feel in your heart that matters."

Each child coped in different ways. Bob felt very angry. He and Alan had shared a special bond. They seemed to think alike and shared the same approach to life. Leslie cried a lot. She and Alan were both hard-headed, and she had lost her sparring partner. David seemed dazed. He spent the whole summer building a tree house for his kids. That was his way of working through Alan's death.

David and Sandra expected their second child that summer. I knew the fact that Poppa would never see their child weighed heavily on both of their hearts. Sandra began labor on August 4, 1995. It rained all day. As a family, we hovered somewhere between feeling excited and feeling sad. Just as the baby was born, the rain stopped, the sun peeked out, and a vibrant rainbow covered the sky. It was so vivid it almost hurt my eyes. David looked at Alana, his newborn daughter, and said, "There's Poppa; he's with us."

Another difficult loss came with the death of my housekeeper, Jessie Mae Royal, who was like a mother to me. In fact, I lived with her for twenty-seven years—longer than I lived with my own mother!

Jessie came to me right after David's birth. After a horse-riding accident at eighteen, then another fall while riding, then a ruptured disk, my back was in bad shape. During labor with David, I pinched a nerve and couldn't even walk.

The doctor sent a nurse named Perky to take care of me and the little ones at home. Perky, a short black woman wearing a red cap with a buckle, appeared at the door, looked me up and down, and said, "You get in bed. Give me that baby." I did as I was told.

Perky brought Jessie along with her as a house-keeper. I came to rely on Jessie's solid presence around the house, and I relished Perky's fried chicken and biscuits. Both women had a tender way with the babies. In the year it took for my leg to recover, Perky and Jessie managed my whole house. After a while, I didn't really need Perky, but she stayed on, and Jessie stayed longer.

Both Jessie and I were quiet. Occasionally I would rant about something Alan did and Jessie would say, "That's a good man, a good man. You're a very lucky lady." Or I'd complain about Bobby or Leslie, and Jessie would say, "Those are nice kids. You do a good job." Relieved, I'd give Jessie a hug.

I wanted to pick Jessie up from the bus stop on snowy days. "No, no," she'd say, "Mrs. Miller, you're not gonna do that. You just stay in bed and I'll get there." I would try to figure out where Jessie was and get her. Sometimes I missed her, some-times I found her.

In 1990, Jessie contracted lung cancer. She arrived every day but did very little, maybe making a bed or wiping up a bathroom. I knew Jessie felt sick but she didn't want to admit it. When I asked if she was OK, she'd say, "Yes, Mrs. Miller, I am just a little tired."

Her funeral was the only time I ever really cried. Jessie had asked that my children be pallbearers, and we were the only white people in a sea of black faces. Everybody knew us. People kept saying, "You're Leslie, you're Bobby, you're David, we know all about you." They made us feel like part of the family. Everybody started crying and wailing, and so did I. In fact, I couldn't stop crying.

I don't know why I could cry at Jessie's funeral. Every other time I've suffered a loss, I have been unable to release the tears I felt. My pattern is to mourn deeply—and silently. Every molecule in my body might ache with sorrow, but I will gather myself together and focus on something else. This ability to compartmentalize is a survival skill I learned from childhood.

I followed that pattern when my mother was diagnosed with cancer. There was nobody in Oklahoma City to take care of her, since my father had died and my uncle who lived with her had just passed away. My sister Judy and I decided to take turns caring for her, two weeks on and two weeks off, so our mother would never be alone.

I was in the midst of planning the Evening of Caring, the first big fundraiser for the Day of Caring. So I worked on the event, flew to Oklahoma City to stay with my mother, returned after two weeks, and picked up planning again. A group of dedicated men and women ensured that the Evening of Caring proceeded without a hitch, while I switched mechanically from nursemaid to event organizer.

After Alan's death, people would ask, "How are you doing?" and I'd say, "OK," even though I was a mess. I think sometimes our deepest feelings are so powerful we can't release them, for fear we'll never regain control. I have so many tears backlogged that it's a wonder I don't gurgle when I walk.

We all cope with loss in different ways. I hold my losses inside, but I also cradle tender memories, joy and hope. The love I feel from the world—and for it—propels me along even when I'm wounded. I'm not only a cancer survivor, I'm a life survivor.

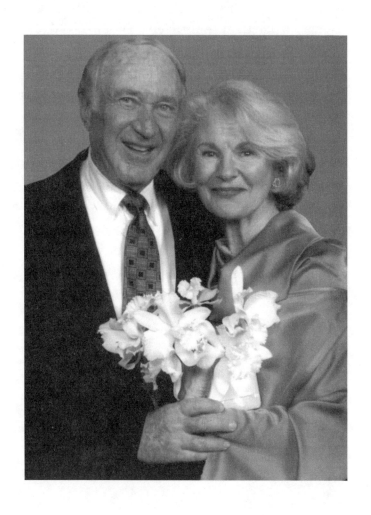

Skip and me at our wedding

A New Love

About a year after I lost Alan, I started dating. Friends would send me off on blind dates, most of which were pleasant enough but never amounted to anything. The bar scene turned into a joke. After a single outing with a group of divorcees, I decided I disliked the whole experience. I had heard about the bar scene being a meat market and it really was.

I didn't have any better luck on my own. I had married so young, I never dated much. I decided it would be glamorous to go to a bar by myself and order a drink. I knew that even one glass of wine would set me on my nose, but I thought I could order a Coke and still feel sophisticated. I thought, *I'm never going to tell anybody I did this.* I drove down Colfax Avenue and found a quiet, pleasant-looking bar. I walked in, perched on a red barstool, and ordered a Coke. As I sat there, sipping my soda, I felt very proud of myself. Then I smoked a cigarette (another adventure).

As I rose to leave, my knee buckled and I fell to the floor. My leg had fallen asleep! The pain shot through my ankle, but all I could think was, *Oh no, I'm going to have to call my kids and tell them what I was doing.* I didn't know anyone in the bar, and I didn't want to. I hobbled to a pay phone, called Bob, and said, "I'm fine but, you know, I had a little accident and I kind of got off a chair and my leg was asleep and now I've hurt my ankle. I can't drive my car. Will you come pick me up?"

"Where are you, Mother?" he asked.

I took a deep breath. "Jack's Bar on Colfax."

"What are you doing there?

"Please don't ask me any questions. Just come get me."

"OK," Bob said, perplexed.

The man who owned the bar worried I would sue him and kept asking, "What can I do? What can I do?" Looking back, I realize I could have asked him to take me to the hospital initially and my kids wouldn't have known. But I waited for my son to appear. He walked in the door, put his arm around my shoulder, and said, "Mother, what got into you?"

I understood what the scene must have looked like: a widow, drinking alone and falling down, spraining an ankle. Everyone would probably think I was drunk. Fortunately the bartender spoke up. "She just had a Coke," he said, leaving me with a tiny piece of dignity. That was my first and last foray into a bar alone.

The awkwardness of dating continued even when I began seeing Skip, the man who became my second husband. Friends asked me to dinner and, a little later, they called and said, "Would you mind if Skip Sigman goes with us?" He was too shy to ask me himself.

I said, "Of course I wouldn't." Alan and I had known Skip and his wife for years. Skip had been divorced for almost twenty-five years when he began seeing me. My friends and Skip grew up together, so when we arrived at the steak house the three of them talked incessantly about old times. I sat there while they reminisced, listening to who went to school where and who they used to date and what parties they attended. Perturbed, I thought, *This is the most boring evening I've ever been through.*

My friends asked if I would mind if Skip took me home. In the driveway I said to him, "That was the most boring evening I ever had in my whole life. You might have tried to talk to me. I don't bite."

We both laughed. He gave me a friendly peck on the cheek and left. When I walked into the house, I thought, *That takes care of that.*

When he called later to ask me out, I hesitated. But when I thought about it, we had been friends for a long time. Maybe it would be nice to have a friend who socialized in the same circle I did. If we both knew everyone, it would be comfortable. I agreed to see him again, and we started dating regularly, going to movies or taking walks. I found him to be a very sweet, kind man. There was never any agenda with Skip, never anything hidden in what he did.

About a year later, Skip said something about traveling together. I replied, "I have five grandsons, Skip, and if I'm going to travel with anybody, I don't care who they are, I'm going to have to be married, because that's just the way I feel it should be."

He said, "OK."

A little surprised at his immediate acquiescence, I said, "I think we need to talk about this." We decided it would be a good idea if we both indulged in a little therapy to help us ease into the marriage. I knew Skip felt nervous about getting married again. I never asked what happened with his first marriage, but I could see it would take him awhile to trust me. Sometimes Skip seemed like a wounded bird.

In counseling, we took steps toward being honest with each other. We found it difficult to compromise, although neither really wanted to change the other. For instance, Skip loved going out to dinner every single night and I hated it. I wanted to stay home and cook seven days a week. Things like that were hard to work out. After so many years alone, it took awhile for Skip to realize he needed to consult someone. In the beginning, he often made spontaneous plans for dinner or a trip without even asking me.

I drove him crazy with my planning. He knew that if we received an invitation to a wedding or party, I would buy the gift before he even wrote an RSVP. He used to kid me about Thanksgiving, because I set the table two weeks early.

When we finally decided to marry, Skip suggested we find a justice of the peace.

"No, we are not going to do that," I said. "What we're going to do is have a wedding, and all our children and grandchildren are going to be attendants." Both families were delighted to see us so happy. Leslie, a party planner, took over all the arrangements, from finding my dress to selecting flowers. It seemed like I was the daughter and she was the mother. We both enjoyed it.

We married at our country club, with Leslie along with Skip's son Jim standing up for us. Skip wandered around in a daze during preparations and looked absolutely petrified at the beginning of the ceremony. I felt more confident. I knew exactly what I wanted, and I got it. I wanted a friend, someone to talk to and go out with. It's a world for two people. You can survive as a woman alone, but it is much more fun when you are two.

For our honeymoon, we took a little cruise, followed by a visit to South Carolina to meet a group of Skip's old friends. The group, rowdy and fun, short-sheeted our bed the first night. I thought, *These people are wonderful. But this isn't what you're supposed to do on your honeymoon, is it?* I came to realize that when I married Skip, I married all of his friends. It seemed like everyone he ever met became a lifelong friend.

We also needed to mesh households. Skip sold his house, and I sold mine. I had lived there thirty-seven years. The day I moved out wrenched my heart. I raised my children there. I made strawberry and raspberry jelly from the bushes in the back yard. I watched countless birds swirl through the grape vines. I could barely force myself to close the door and move on. Yet I knew I couldn't stay. I needed to make a new life.

Because of differing sales dates, I moved into Skip's house for a week before the wedding, and I felt so embarrassed about being under the same roof that I snuck in and out. A week after we returned from our honeymoon, we moved into a small apartment in Cherry Creek. Neither one of us ever believed we would love living there, but we became attached to the area. A year later, we looked at a condo being built next door.

The place seemed perfect, except it had three floors. No way was I moving into a house without an elevator. Skip never planned on getting old and needing an elevator. He hadn't spent money for a long time, and all of a sudden there he was, buying a new place and furnishings. He said, "Everything costs so much money!"

I replied, "You know, that's what happens when you get married and you take on a new life. You have to buy a dishwasher. You have to buy a chair and a table and we have to put in an elevator."

We argued for a week. It looked like we would divorce before we were really married. I got my way, though. Thank God we installed the elevator, because we both ended up using the damn thing.

Skip did push me to have the kind of fun I wasn't used to. We took off for rides in the mountain. We visited Florida, enjoying boat rides and walks. We had the most fun. He helped me relax and enjoy myself.

When Skip turned seventy, he and I joined another couple for a Mediterranean cruise. While on board, I developed the flu. The doctor insisted I go to a hospital in Civitavecchia, the port city of Rome, so Skip and I packed our clothes and trundled into an ambulance. When we arrived at the 19th century hospital furnished only with tiny cots, no one spoke English. I knew I was dehydrated but didn't know how to tell the staff. *If that doctor on the boat had just given me an I.V., I'd be fine*, I thought.

They wheeled me to a treatment room while Skip dealt with the receptionist. Then Skip couldn't find me in the hospital. He tried to talk with the staff, but the language barrier was too great. He even tried wandering the halls, peering in rooms, but never found me. I didn't see him for almost two whole days.

While Skip grew frantic, I felt tickled because it was such a funny experience. I decided Skip had returned to the boat, so I made the best of the situation. The building itself felt ancient and imposing. The nurses wore big, tall hats like I had seen in movies. I never felt scared; instead, I found the whole situation amusing. I would stick out my arm and poke at it, trying to convey that I needed an I.V. The Italians, concerned about me, obviously tried their best to help. Sandwiched between two little ladies who spoke nothing but Italian, I never had so much fun!

On the second day without Skip, feeling rehydrated and much refreshed, I kept saying, "I want to go home." The doctor came in, listened to my heart, shook his head, and walked out. A woman who spoke a little English told me my blood pressure was high and the doctor refused to release me.

Shortly thereafter, Skip poked his head in the door. He looked like he might cry when he saw me. "I thought you were dead," he croaked. "I couldn't find you anywhere. Nobody would tell me where you were." By then the adventure was wearing down, and I was never so glad to see anyone in my life. My guardian angel stood in that doorway. He wanted to find the doctor, but I said, "No, don't leave me! We might get separated again."

Both of us were anxious to leave, and Skip tried to find someone to authorize my release. He couldn't.

Finally we just walked out and caught the boat in another port.

I felt charmed with Skip, as though the world waited like a giant surprise party. I finally enjoyed the companionship I had sought. The two of us floated along, secure in our love, expecting a long and happy marriage.

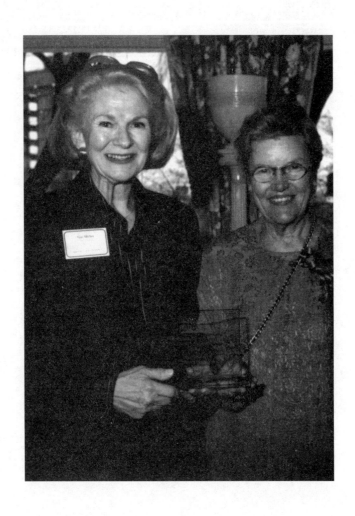

Receiving the Bea Romer Women's
Health Leadership Award

Feeling Fragile

In 2002, I suffered a mild stroke. It began with a TIA (Transient Ischemic Attack). I stayed in a hospital for a few days, disoriented and walking very slowly, but the symptoms faded. Then I experienced another TIA, but not as bad as the first.

The third episode was a full-blown stroke. As he left for an appointment, Skip said to me, "The newspaper didn't come this morning. I'm going to go get one before I leave." When he returned, I was standing at the sink. I muttered, "I have a terrible pain in my head," and started to fall. Skip knew right away what had happened and rushed me to the hospital.

In the car, I couldn't move my right side or even talk. I glanced over at Skip's jovial face, now drawn with worry. How lucky for me that he decided to get a newspaper, because otherwise I would have been alone and unable to call for help. Fortunately, too, Skip decided to go to the hospital immediately, because if a stroke victim is diagnosed within three hours and given medication to dissolve the clot, the chances of long-term damage are minimized.

At the hospital, I received the medication. Then, unable to speak, I watched Skip and my children hover. They all tried to be cheerful, but I knew they thought I would die. I couldn't reassure them. I could open my mouth, but emitted not one word. I felt sorry for them all, seeing the looks on their faces and not being able to tell them I'd be OK. After about three hours, I felt a return of sensation.

Even with some speech regained, I had trouble concentrating. I experienced double vision in both of my eyes, along with loss of peripheral vision. Just before the stroke I had a cataract removed, which caused some hemorrhaging in my left eye. Of course I lost vision in that eye, and the peripheral vision never returned. I am not able to drive anymore. I can't see if anything is coming from the side, and I cannot read a street sign.

I remained in the hospital four days, then transferred downstairs to rehabilitation for two weeks, regaining some strength and relearning what I had lost. After my release, I went to an outpatient center to learn to walk again. It seemed like I had to tell my legs how to move. If I came to a step, my leg didn't know what to do. The rehabilitation therapist would say, "You have to talk to your leg," as if talking to my leg would make it go. For a while I used a walker, which I hated, and then a cane, which I also hated. I felt like I was a hundred thousand years old.

To my amazement, the rehabilitation center treated more than just old people. Young people, in their thirties and forties, had suffered strokes much worse than mine. Some sat in wheelchairs that they probably would never leave. I felt particular compassion for one young girl, an artist who had been in a motorcycle wreck with no helmet on. She had been at the rehabilitation center every day for four years. When I looked at her and the other young people, my heart broke for them. At the same time, I told myself, *That's not me. I'm not going to be here for the rest of my life.* Being at rehabilitation motivated me to push myself toward wellness.

I learned to read again, too. I could read a paragraph but couldn't quite gather the whole of it, the words fluttering in the air like bits of confetti. I have great difficulty reading a whole book because of my eyes. Most of my "reading" is done on tapes. At the university where I study, a program for the disabled puts all of my textbooks on tape free of charge so I can keep up.

The loss of independence from my stroke is one of the hardest things I have ever dealt with. Thankfully, from the beginning I received lots of help getting around. Skip never told me no, no matter what I asked of him. He was always there with a smile on his face and a hug. My children and their spouses, as well as my grandchildren, lift my spirits because they are always there to help me.

I learned how fragile life is. In two seconds the whole world can change. One of my fears now is further losing my independence. The medication I take that thins my blood to prevent another stroke also makes my body bruise easily. I look like somebody beat me up. To keep in shape, I walk, stretch and lift weights.

After the stroke, I knew I needed to hand the Day of Caring reins over to someone else and concentrate on getting well. I couldn't attend everyday meetings because I simply was not strong enough. So I stepped back. If I wanted the project to go on without me—and I came close to not making it—I needed to let people step in and take over. Part of me wanted to think, *Oh, without me it couldn't keep going.* But I never truly believed that the event would falter when I stepped back from it. I saw it marching into the future.

Elise Spain understood how I felt and never failed to call me and consult about decisions. "Should we add a seminar?" "Should we sell table space?" Elise could make those decisions, but she chose to keep me informed. I will always be grateful to her for protecting my feelings.

It was a tough year, though—not for the Day of Caring, but for me. I didn't know who I was without it. I felt lost. I continued to sit in on the board meetings, and it took a year and half before I could bite my tongue and not say anything. I knew the board entertained new and bright ideas and I needed to respect them. The volunteer force just kept growing.

After I started to feel better, I wanted to jump back in but knew I shouldn't. It was like having a child—you know the child must become independent, but it's so hard to let go. I felt that I *was* the Day of Caring. I kept thinking, *Who am I? Am I anything without the Day of Caring?*

I searched for something to replace it. A few years prior to the stroke, I had met a young Mexican girl who had a bilateral mastectomy. She could not adjust to the loss of both breasts. Her husband and children felt so frightened that they could not help her. She needed help badly but the family was too poor to buy insurance and too rich to qualify for Medicaid. In the end, she killed herself. I swore I would never let that happen again, that someday I would start a free mental health clinic for people like her.

I remembered the promise I made to open a mental health clinic for the uninsured. I knew I needed to have a master's degree in counseling and psychology to open a clinic, so I called my daughter Leslie. She drove me to the University of Colorado at Denver for information. I remember saying, "Leslie, what am I doing? I'm sixty-nine years old and going to start a master's program. I've lost my mind!"

Leslie replied, "It's not going to hurt to go down and find out."

. After I met with the head of the department and discovered all the application paperwork I needed to complete, I thought, *I don't think I can do this.* But of course I did. I filled out all the applications, obtained my school records, and wrote a letter explaining why I wanted to be accepted into the master's program.

When things pile up and I feel overwhelmed, I think I can't go on—and then I go on. Being in class, meeting new people, and having a different focus brought me out of feeling so lost without the Day of Caring. When life whacks you, you have to be strong enough to take the steps toward another life. You have to face that fear and put it behind you.

One day, sitting in the campus cafeteria listening to a textbook on tape, I looked up. Students lounged and chatted, drank coffee and studied quietly. I felt a rush of happiness at being there. The world seemed suddenly full of possibilities.

I realized that, without knowing it, I had grown away from the Day of Caring even before my stroke. Years of listening to the stories of participants, brave and difficult and poignant as they were, had taken its toll. Now I listen to new sounds—the gabble of students, the authoritative voice of a professor, the swirl of ideas in my own mind. Part of me still longs to be head of the Day of Caring, but another part has welcomed my new life.

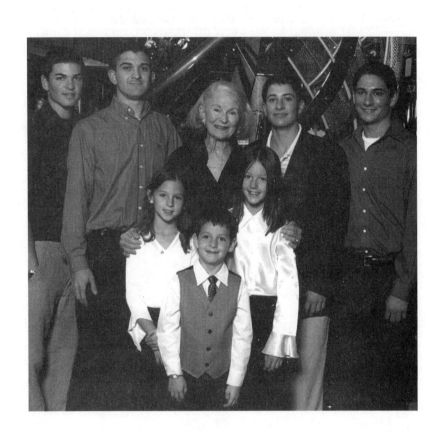

Me and my grandchildren on the Caribbean cruise

ANOTHER GOOD-BYE

In December 2003, Skip and I took my whole family on a cruise to the Caribbean. Fifteen of us boarded ship for a rowdy time together. Skip had a little cough but seemed cheerful throughout the trip. When we docked in Miami, I said, "Let's both go to the doctor for a checkup." The doctor took a chest X-ray of Skip and told us to return home right away. He could see tumors lodged throughout Skip's lungs.

On January 10, 2004, after only six years of marriage, Skip was diagnosed with Stage IV melanoma. The cancer had infiltrated his lungs. After the initial diagnosis, he wouldn't talk about what he felt. He always kept a smile on his face, saying, "I am not going to die!"

Although I tried not to let Skip see, I felt completely distraught. I thought, *I don't want you to die! I don't want to go through this again. I lost one husband, and I don't know if I can bear to go through widowhood again.* We were both afraid. At the same time, we were gentle with one another; I didn't force Skip to talk, but eventually he began to share his worries. He didn't fear dying but he worried about becoming an invalid. I let him talk, listening with my breaking heart. Every once in a while Skip would start to apologize for messing up our lives with his illness. I would say, "I don't care if we have just this time. We've had such fun. It's been a good marriage."

"I love you so much. Thank you for being with me," he'd say.

"I wouldn't be anyplace else, Skip."

Our marriage was one of caring for each other. Through hard times, we both maintained an attitude of putting this difficult situation in a certain place and enjoying whatever life brought in the moment. We both prized a sense of humor. You try not to let the power of an illness consume your whole life. You try to live every day to the fullest and not let the illness ruin the time you have.

I watched Skip go progressively downhill. He underwent radiation and two clinical trials. As long as he thought there was hope, he would consider any treatment. And as long as he kept moving, he could stave off depression. I, too, kept moving, forcing myself to go to school. Once again I dealt with difficult times by focusing on something else.

When I started to obsess about losing him, I would force myself to imagine the worst possible thing that could happen. For me, that would be if my family fell apart, if they fought and yelled and didn't care for me anymore. *Anything else I can cope with*, I told myself.

My children and Skip's children helped me through Skip's illness. My daughter-in-law Sandy understood completely since her own mother was suffering from ovarian cancer. Sandy found it difficult to talk about either situation, but she always gave me a hug and a kiss, saying, "I'm there for you." I knew all of their hearts hurt. They all called daily to check on us. That was life: We could do nothing about it. Around Thanksgiving 2004, Skip started to seriously decline. The doctor said over and over that Skip didn't have a chance. He never gave one good report. Skip felt so determined to keep himself going that it took awhile for him to realize he wasn't going to make it. He loved living, and he would live fully until he died. Basically he did.

In his last couple of months he grew physically weak and hated every single minute of it. He couldn't walk, not even around the front of the house. We never stopped going out to dinner, because he wanted to. His whole life was people. He loved being around people, and they loved him back. Every day the phone would ring at least thirty times, and I would repeat the same account of Skip's health. Finally, I started an email list and once a week wrote a letter to kids, family and friends. It saved my voice and kept everyone up to date.

In November Skip discovered bumps on his head, all melanoma. He underwent another round of radiation so difficult that I wondered if it actually made things worse. He gradually lost all strength. He couldn't hold his pants up any longer, and he had trouble eating. The doctor said it would be a matter of a month or so. In December friends visited, including Skip's best friend from Florida. They came in for New Year's Eve and enjoyed a wonderful visit. My sister and brother-in-law also were there. After they left, Skip deteriorated more.

As I took care of Skip, I learned a valuable, unexpected lesson. I hadn't known how difficult it is to be a caregiver. In my lifetime I have taken care of many people, including models and friends who were dying, but it wasn't the same as caring for someone so close to me. I had always been able to work easily with dying people, talking with them frankly about what needed to be completed, comforting them. When you're doing it for somebody you really love, though, you feel it so deeply that it wears you down. You want to be there for the person you love, but you don't want to be there to watch the suffering. It's a struggle every day.

I would rise in the morning knowing what I would face that day, knowing I would soon lose someone I loved. How could I wear a smile on my face? How could I keep things moving along like normal, when life was not normal and never would be? Leaving to have my hair done, I found it hard to walk out of the house. And once out of the house I didn't want to come back

Skip's suffering affected me so much I could not think straight. I knew and loved him. I knew when he pondered whether or not he would survive. The look on his face resembled that of a hurt little boy whose best toy or puppy had been snatched. His life was being squeezed away. When I saw him struggle to leave a chair, that lost look flashed across his face. With each report from the doctor, I saw the same expression, as though Skip said to me, *Why? Why is this happening to me?* He never spoke those words, but I saw it. At night when we went to bed, we would talk a little bit about him getting worse. But once he left that bedroom, he never talked about dying.

The family never left him alone for a minute. His kids, my kids, we all became one family struggling because someone we loved was dying. We all stayed nearby because we knew Skip felt scared. He started sleeping a lot. On the 14th of January, 2005, the rabbi from the temple visited, along with the cantor from another congregation. I didn't know why they chose that morning to come over but there they were. Skip's son had gone upstairs to help his father dress, and Skip just walked down the stairs and sat down to talk with everyone. He felt a sense of peace, I think, when talking with people.

While the rabbi and cantor sat there, Skip's doctor called to say the latest reports looked very bad. He told me, "You've got to get hospice in there right now, because he's in for a bad, bad time." Skip didn't want hospice, though. A week before, when I had found Skip covered with blood from his skin lesions, I asked a man to come help me bathe and dress Skip. Skip hated it, just hated it.

It sounded like the pain would become unbearable and we needed to start strong medication as soon as possible. When I hung up the phone, I walked upstairs, stood on the porch outside our bedroom, and said, "If there really is a God and you want me to believe, you'll take him now." Then I went back downstairs. The rabbi and cantor left and all Skip's family came over like they did every day.

About 5 p.m. his kids left and my children brought dinner: lo mein, Skip's favorite. They picked him up from the chair so he could sit at the table. He had eaten so little for the past couple of weeks and probably didn't even want the food, but he made a brave effort. He put a bite of lo mein in his mouth, and I heard his throat rattle slightly. I thought he was choking, so I held a napkin to his mouth, but then I realized I was hearing his last breaths. Alan's death flashed across my mind. It felt the same. My mind shifted into slow motion: *This is the second time this has happened to me.*

Alan gave me a kiss goodnight, turned over, and died.
Skip is dying at the dinner table.

My three youngest grandchildren were sitting right there, along with David and Sandy. When Skip's throat began rattling, they looked spooked. David said, "That noise is God coming to get Skip." Sandy took the kids to the other room. I tried to call Skip's doctor but couldn't reach him. David and I looked at Skip's immobile face. I asked, "David, do you think he's gone?"

"Mom, I think he is."

I called 911. When the paramedics arrived, they hovered over Skip, who lay on the floor. I yelled, "Don't resuscitate him!"

"Do you have a medical directive, ma'am?" one paramedic asked.

"No, I don't think so."

"I'm sorry, but unless you have a medical directive in the house, the emergency staff by law has to resuscitate."

I thought of the pain Skip would face if the paramedics managed to pull him back from death. At that point, Skip's doctor walked in and said, "Leave him alone, don't try to resuscitate him."

"Thank you," I said gratefully. I looked at Skip's tall, now frail body lying on the floor. I whispered to him, *You don't have to go through that, Skip.* I was prepared for Skip's death, yet unprepared. I want to tell everyone now: Keep your medical directive in your home.

Laurie, our silky terrier and princess of the family, never left Skip's side during his last few weeks. She used to bark so loudly that people thought she was a much larger dog. If you couldn't see her tiny body emitting those huge barks, you actually might be scared. For the month before Skip died, Laurie stopped barking at anybody, instead keeping a silent vigil over Skip. The night he died, she sat right by his body as the paramedics prepared to transport him. She never left his side until they took him from the house.

From that point, events rolled on. I knew what I needed to do, getting everybody through shiva, having the funeral on Sunday. I was amazed by all the people in the house the two weeks before and after Skip's death. A continuous stream of well-wishers shuffled through, bringing food and paying their respects. It seemed overwhelming. I mostly remember the number of people who said things like, "Skip was a wonderful man. He was never as happy as when he was married to you. You were a very special couple."

A new school semester was scheduled to start a week later, and I wondered whether or not I should begin. I decided it would be good for me, and it was. It gave me one day a week to focus on something concrete. In a stroke of luck, the course I registered for was "Methods in Group Counseling." For a whole semester I had to be part of the group process. It gave me a chance to share my burdens.

When I think about Skip, my heart is full of tears. I just don't know how to force the tears from my eyes. I miss him, of course. I miss the wonderful times we shared together. Ours was a marriage not of deep romance but of fun and companionship. We were soul mates, because he understood how I felt about the problems I had, and I understood about the problems he had, too. We shared a good marriage.

I have never believed in mourning. Skip's children, my children, and I gave whatever we had to give while he lived. We made every moment of his life as good as we could. People have to realize that today is today, and you let somebody know you love them today. When they're gone, they're gone and they don't know what you're doing afterward. You have to move on.

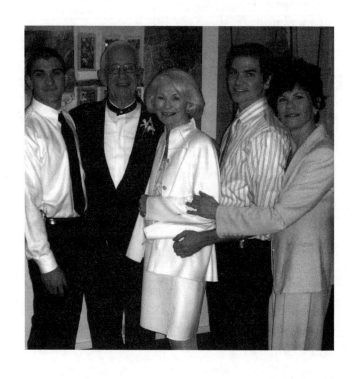

*Bride and Groom, married January 1, 2006.
grandson Nathan, Harold, me, grandson Jeremy,
and daughter Leslie*

SELF-ESTEEM—
AN INSIDE JOB

I displayed a sticker on my car for years that read "Self-esteem – An Inside Job." The dictionary defines self-esteem as pride in oneself. You have also heard, I am sure, that you cannot love anyone else until you have learned to love yourself. I think these two sayings relate not just to me but to all of us. I don't think you can have self-esteem unless you love yourself.

Self-esteem is a tiny voice in all of us that makes a day fabulous or terrible. It can make our relationship with our family and friends wonderful or awful. It's a choice. It is easier to live when that tiny voice tells us that we are OK. We can accept others and situations better when we are not looking at the dark side of people, situations or ourselves.

For instance, I could shout my feelings every morning. I could scream: Why has all this happened? Why the sexual abuse, why cancer and the loss of a breast, why a stroke? Why did I have to lose my husbands? But screaming and crying wouldn't help. Nothing can entirely remove the pain I've felt in my life. My kids, my husbands, my friends, everyone I know could do everything in the world to be good and kind—and they are—but the heartache inside me never disappears.

I accept it. I accept myself, even if I wish I were different. I wish I could cry. In fact, I set a goal during my group counseling classes to cry. I never achieved it. My eyes might moisten, my nose would run, but no tears spilled out. It became an ongoing joke to my group and then to my kids. Now, if I have a runny nose, my children say, "Mom's crying again."

Instead of crying, I take action. The sadness doesn't impede me, it doesn't stop me from going to meetings or feeding the dog. I look around to see where I can make a difference in other people's lives, filling the cavern inside with activity: parenting, modeling, nursing, the Day of Caring, and now counseling those in need. I put that pain away on a daily basis and just get on with my life. Rather than being angry and hating everything around me, or trying to escape through pills or alcohol, I take that energy and put it to work helping the world I live in become a better place.

Besides raising three wonderful children, my greatest accomplishment is the Day of Caring for Breast Cancer Awareness. When I am at the Day of Caring and I look out into the crowd of a thousand men and women, all ages, colors, and different ethnic backgrounds, my heart swells with pride. Everyone in that room sees the Day of Caring as a place where age and ethnicity don't matter. Participants are sisters and brothers who have shared a life experience and are struggling to go on with their lives. They are all coming together to support each other, and by sharing their stories they help themselves, mentally and physically. The education we provide at the Day of Caring gives everyone a chance to regain control of their lives.

The dream I am pursuing now is a master's degree in counseling and psychology at the University of Colorado at Denver. I have one more year of classes, then a practicum and internship. With school, I feel a whole new life awaits me. It gives me a way to work toward my new mission, counseling for the indigent, homeless and uninsured.

All my life I have felt a particular compassion for the homeless. I know that I've enjoyed good fortune in my life. I've been able to access help when I was sick. So I have great compassion for those who don't have that opportunity.

Once when modeling in downtown Denver, I passed a corner where a bag lady sat. Something about the woman's face made me stop and say, "Do you know you are beautiful?" She didn't reply, but later, upon seeing a broadcast of the show I had done that day, she called the television station to tell her

story. She said she'd been sitting on the corner think-
ing about committing suicide. When I spoke to her,
it was the first time anyone had shown her kindness
in a very long time. I cherish that story. So often we
don't hear about the effects of our actions.

I entered my master's program with the idea of
opening a free mental health clinic. I could charge
a dollar an hour for somebody who needs it, or go
into homeless shelters. Many retired therapists and
social workers have told me they'd love to participate
in such a program, volunteering a few hours a week.

I have already talked to foundations, mental
health facilities, hospitals, and universities about
their programs. Much to my surprise, I found that
low-cost therapy is available and several agencies
offer pro bono services. The problem is no one
knows about these agencies. So for the moment I am
going to finish school and put together a resource
book for distribution to mental health agencies
and nonprofits. I would also like to have a mental
health component under the umbrella of the Day of
Caring. It's a big undertaking but many people out
there understand what I want to do and will guide
me in the right direction.

People have asked me, "Oh my God, how did you
do this? How come you're still smiling?" I look at them
and say, "There's nothing I'm doing that you couldn't
do if you faced the same circumstances." Maybe some

people will lose a husband and that ends their lives. Or they suffer from sexual abuse and relive that the rest of their lives. They'll have cancer and live cancer the rest of their days. But for the most part, people possess a really strong spirit that can enable them to survive these things. So my spirituality is the belief in human beings and the values that guide them. I think that is God.

My religious beliefs are uniquely my own. I know that there's a God somewhere. I don't know who or what he is, probably somebody deep in my heart. I don't think he's responsible for anything, I don't think he guides anything. I believe in the human spirit. I believe in people and the ability they have to survive. I believe in helping people do what they can for themselves. I hold a deep respect for what people do as they struggle through life and keep going.

My advice to women who have been abused: Believe in yourself. Your feelings are real and nobody needs to put up with that. You're too good a human being to have this happen. I know it's easy to stop believing in yourself, but you have to keep seeing the good and work from that point. If you're abused you think you have done something wrong so you deserve everything you're getting. But let me tell you, nobody has the right to abuse another person. The abuser is always wrong. I encourage victims to find something in themselves to believe in—whether it's giving birth, or obtaining an education, or knowing how to embroider. Look at the good things you've done in your life and build on those qualities.

For people who are feeling isolated, I encourage you to step away from those feelings and do something. If your kids haven't called for a while, and you think, *They don't care about me*, pick up the phone and say, "Kids, I'm having dinner. Come over." Don't just sit there and feel bad because they haven't called you fourteen times a day. Think enough of yourself to step in and say, "This is what I want from you, I want to be with you."

It is possible to find fulfilling relationships at any stage of life. I never expected to fall in love again, much less marry. But on New Year's Day 2006, I married Harold Cohen, a man I had known for years. We dated briefly two years after Alan died. After a few months, Harold kissed me, not our usual peck on the cheek, but a real kiss. I felt my mind and body respond—a scary situation. Because of my experience with my father, I was not capable of being a good sexual partner. I wasn't ready to allow any romance or sexuality in my life. Alan and Skip both understood how scared I was, and they never pushed me. I felt safe with them.

I had eight years to think about that kiss and the idea of a romantic relationship. Harold called when he heard Skip was dying. Harold's wife had died similarly, and he wanted to offer help and advice. Skip passed in January 2005, and in August Harold asked me to lunch. After his call, I sat at my kitchen table, looking at chickadees flit onto the birdfeeder outside the window. I was seventy-one years old. I could accept my life the way it was, or I could try to become the woman I wanted to be. I went to lunch with Harold, who gazed at me tenderly but with a gleam in his eye. On a trip to the bookstore I bought one of those garish yellow instructional guides: *Sex for Dummies.*

When Harold asked me to marry him, I told him there was a possibility I could lose my eyesight. He said, "It doesn't matter. You know I don't hear well. So I will be your eyes and you can be my ears."

I am not sure that one can have a romance like this when both people are young, raising children, and working to succeed in careers. In a way, a romance at this time of life is very selfish. Harold and I can focus entirely on each other, spending hours talking and making love. We draw on the best part of our marriages before, remembering our other spouses, not trying to replace them, but grateful for the experiences that brought us here. I am awestruck at having found love again. I'm having one of the best times of my life!

For my children and grandchildren, and as a matter of fact for everyone, my advice is geared toward courage. Always leave yourselves open for good things that come along in your lives. Don't be afraid to try. Don't waste time on the past; deal with what you have to and find some way to put the past to rest. Sure, it pops up, but don't let it ruin the rest of your life. Open yourselves to the future. The past affects us, but don't stay there. It's important to move on.

I am grateful for my life experiences, especially doing work with the Day of Caring. If I died today, I could truly say that I had everything that any person would ever want in their life, bad and good alike. The fact that I've been able to help change destructive thinking and leave an imprint on people's lives means everything to me. My experiences gave me wisdom to draw on when I helped others. I think that is what they call making lemons into lemonade.

Maybe I was destined to follow this path in life. One might see in my story the hand of Fate, grooming me from infanthood to be hyperaware of my body and self-esteem. Or one might see an example of Free Will, a woman faced with difficult choices who finally triumphs. I myself don't know which it is. Whatever one may see in my life, I have learned to respect and love myself for who I am regardless of my shortcomings. I realize that until you respect the inside of you, you cannot have self-esteem.

And that's my story so far. I appreciate who I've become. I'm not a frightened child any more, or just a pretty face. I'm not a woman with missing parts. I'm a loving and loved mother, grandmother, friend, and wife. I can look in the mirror and smile as I see that I haven't been completely worn down by life. I laugh as I think, *I'm tougher than I look!*

RESOURCES

DAY OF CARING FOR BREAST
CANCER AWARENESS
Phone 303-239-3434
Email: info@dayofcaringonline.org
Web: www.dayofcaringonline.org

CANCER INFORMATION AND
COUNSELING LINE (CICL)
Phone 303-239-3422 or 800-525-3777
This service of AMC Cancer Research Center
offers cancer information, support from trained
counselors, and services in English and Spanish.

AMERICAN CANCER SOCIETY NATIONAL
CANCER INFORMATION CENTER
Phone 800-227-2345
Information and support 24 hours a day, 7 days
a week. A breast cancer survivor will answer the
phone live on Tuesdays from 11 a.m. to 3 p.m. EST.
Any other time, leave a message and a breast cancer
survivor will return your call within 24 hours.

BEYOND BREAST CANCER
SURVIVORS' HELPLINE
(American Cancer Society)
Phone 888-753-5222

ROCKY MOUNTAIN CANCER
INFORMATION SERVICE
Phone 800-422-6237
This service of the National Cancer Institute
offers information in English and Spanish about
prevention, detection, and treatment options, as
well as referrals to other support organizations.

SUSAN G. KOMEN BREAST
CANCER FOUNDATION
Phone 800-462-9273
Talk about breast cancer issues with a
survivor. Services in English and Spanish.

Y-ME NATIONAL BREAST
CANCER ORGANIZATION
Phone 800-221-2141 (English),
800-986-9505 (Spanish)
Talk with a trained peer counselor who
is also a breast cancer survivor. When
possible, caller is matched with a counselor
who has a similar diagnosis.

JEWISH FAMILY SERVICE
COUNSELING LINE
Phone 303-597-7777

COPING WITH CANCER MAGAZINE
Reading for people whose lives have
been touched by cancer.
Web: www.copingmag.com